25 Months

A Memoir

LINDA McK. STEWART

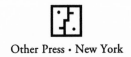

Other Press · New York

"Burnt Norton" from FOUR QUARTERS by T. S. Eliot, copyright 1936 by Harcourt, Inc. and renewed 1964 by T. S. Eliot, reprinted by permission of the publisher.

Copyright © 2004 Linda McK. Stewart

Production Editor: Robert D. Hack

Designer: Natalya Balnova

This book was set in Caslon 540 Roman by Alpha Graphics of Pittsfield, NH.

10 9 8 7 6 5 4 3 2 1

Library of Congress Cataloging-in-Publication Data

Mck. Stewart, Linda.
    25 months : a memoir / by Linda Mck. Stewart.
        p. cm.
    Includes bibliographical references.
    ISBN 1-59051-130-1 (hardcover : alk. paper)
    1. Mck. Stewart, Linda.   2. Caregivers–Biography.   3. Alzheimer's disease–Patients–Home care.   4. Alzheimer's disease–Patients–Family relationships.
I. Title: Twenty-five months.   II. Title.
    RC523.2.M393 2004
    362.196'831–dc22

                                                          2004002654

FOR MY FAMILY, WITH GRATITUDE

Special thanks to
the Vermont Studio Center, Johnson, Vermont

Time present and time past
Are both perhaps present in time future,
And time future contained in time past.
If all time is eternally present
All time is unredeemable.

—T. S. Eliot,
Four Quartets

PROLOGUE

Four windows form the headboard of our bed. A straggle of trees, the marsh, and then the river. Milky moonlight floods our pillows. Behind me his knees fit perfectly into the soft caps of my bent legs. His chin rests easily on the top of my head. His arm crosses my body in that little valley just below my ribs. The soles of my feet lie flat against his shins. Am I awake or asleep? Maybe both. His thumb explores the back of my hand, pauses on my fourth finger, and idly turns the gold band there. Time and the cool of the night have deepened the groove and the ring turns easily. Above me his breath is warm in my ear.

"Marry me," he murmurs.

Dream or joke? His words, my torpor, merge to pursue me through the shallows of sleep. But already I'm far ahead, sinking into the deep. In the morning the moon and his words have vanished . . . forgotten. It seems.

1

IMPRESSION: . . . On the short test of mental status, he scored well within the normal range statistically giving him at most around a 10% chance of having a dementing illness such as Alzheimer's disease.

Dr. X

That last day before the beginning was a blue and gold Sunday, cool and clear, the kind of perfection only October can confer. We attended a community picnic, a tacit farewell to bare feet, to shirtsleeves, and to all the insouciance of life in balmy weather.

We were tossed, Jack and I, along with a handful of our peer group, into this hilltop gathering like seasoning, just a pinch but not too much, because the day belonged to the young, two or three dozen parents, kids in tow. On the grass in front of the old turn-of-the-century clubhouse, Frisbee-tossing fathers in khakis and sneakers were in full command. Leggy, summer-tanned mothers, still coiffed in the shining hair of girlhood, took their ease on the wide wooden steps, casually watchful of their tyrannical toddlers playing on the lawn beyond. Smoke from a couple of cooking grills drifted up through flamboyant foliage as the self-appointed chefs stood around taking orders and exchanging the latest inanities harvested from their weekday 9 to 5 existences.

Ours was a comfortable community. Not chic, just comfortable. A good public school system was amply funded by murderous property taxes. Kids could begin sailing in the River Rats when they were eight. On Sunday afternoon, year round, there were sailboat races, open to anyone who could cinch a line or trim a sail. The public library would obligingly procure any title and make it available for two weeks with a two weeks renewal option, a privilege that went a long way toward keeping the family's book-buying budget under control. In winter, until global warming spoiled the fun, there was ice boating on the river. In summer the epicenter of life moved to an uncrowded beach, lately tripled in size by a beach replenishment program that, residents never tired of gleefully reminding one another, was entirely covered by state and federal funding.

For the most part domesticity was housed in hard-to-heat Victorian houses with wraparound porches. Never intended for year-round living, they were designed for the twentieth century's first quarter, when Irish or southern immigrants were grateful for Thursdays and every other Sunday, along with room and board, minimal salary, and the privilege of being called part of the family. As prized as alcoves and window seats, holly trees and ancient lilacs was a view, of cove, inlet, river curve, marshland, or, for a fortunate few, the open Atlantic. Golf was big but so was tennis, plenty of Har-Tru courts and eighteen pristine grass courts at a club that proudly called itself the oldest tennis club in America. On a summer afternoon passing motorists often paused to take in the sheer aesthetics of the scene: all the courts in play and every player in white, dazzling against the perfection of the emerald turf, a spectacle lifted straight from *Town & Country* circa 1910.

So much pleasant living was financed either by "old money" or by the fallout from long hours in the canyons of lower Manhattan. Many commuted to and from work by double-hulled ferries, a pleasant journey of under an hour. For those still clinging to lower rungs of the economic ladder, there was bus and train service that was occasionally awful but usually not bad.

A sprinkling of scientists and engineers, courtesy of several nearby high-tech corporations, nicely offset all those up-and-coming financial whiz kids, as did a slate of M.D.'s , their imported sports cars easily spotted in the parking area of any local event.

As in most weekend gatherings, Jack was not so easily categorized. His thirty-four years as an editor at *The New York Times,* and his postretirement work as a literary agent and editor of a monthly Harvard newsletter put him in a niche of his own. To the younger generation the very idea of spending one's entire career with a single organization, working your way up, was so quaint as to be almost laughable. Laughable too was the paper's prevailing pay scale during those years, as was the nonindexed pension on which he and I had been living quite happily in the five years since his retirement.

But still, among the young, Jack was something of a favorite. They relished his quirky, irreverent view of the world, more socialist than Democrat, more skeptic than believer. They quoted him, usually with affection, often with incredulity:

"Do away with the CIA? Come on, Jack, I know you're kidding!" or

"Legalize drugs? All drugs? You're not really serious, are you?"

He was unfailingly generous with his time when a friend or acquaintance approached him, manuscript in hand, asking him if he'd "give it a read" and advise what step, if any, should be taken next. Like an original Currier and Ives he was viewed with respectful appreciation. Beyond that, he had earned a toehold in the affections of the community by virtue of a God-given, Harvard-honed talent with a tennis racquet. At Andover and later at Harvard, where he tutored laggards and waited on tables to retain his scholarship, he took to the game with a delight that even now, more than half a century later, was dimmed hardly at all. Many a player half his age had taken him on in singles, courteous, deferential, keenly aware of the arthritic knees that kept the old gent from dashing hither and yon. Then, just beyond the point of no return, the challenger would find, alas too late, that the old gent was killing him with deadly slices, drop shots, lobs, volleys, and a wicked southpaw corkscrew serve.

That Sunday, buttoned into an old Harris tweed jacket, Jack was content to enjoy the surrounding scene from an ancient wicker armchair out on the lawn, his heels propped atop an overturned bucket. Free of any domestic responsibilities, I too was happy doing nothing more constructive than lounging on an old mothy blanket, soaking up the last of the season's sunshine. All around the air crackled with energy generated by laughter and chatter, adult banter, and the delight of children at play. Squinting through my eyelashes I could see a far-off minuscule flotilla of white cruise ships departing New York harbor and moving, left to right along the horizon, heading no doubt for warmer southern waters. Closer in, triangles of sail skittered back and forth across the bay like water bugs. Turned in upon myself, I hovered lazily in some inviolate space, neither of the moment nor aspiring to anything beyond.

Behind me, above me, I only half-listened to an ongoing semi-silly discussion. Bruce Anderson was a young commercial real estate magnate. His undoubted success still seemed to leave him time aplenty in which to head up fund-raisers for conservative political organizations, manage a Little League team, and make the rounds of New England anchorages in summer and prime ski slopes in winter. A true mover and shaker. Now sprawled on the grass beside Jack's chair, he was gnawing at a subject in which Jack took little interest: the recent sale in a depressed market of our lower Manhattan loft where for ten years we'd lived contentedly Monday to Friday.

"If only you'd consulted me," Bruce said, only half kidding.

"And if I had, what would you have advised?"

"I think I'd have said, sit tight. Hang on. Six months more would have made a lot of difference."

"Mm-m-m."

"Well, you must admit, selling at twice what you got, that wouldn't be so bad now would it?"

"Maybe. Maybe not. I just don't know."

"Don't know! I'm not believing this."

"No," said Jack. "Of course you're right. I should have waited. Six months and I could have sold for twice what we got? Is that right?"

"Absolutely."

"Honey, did you hear that?" With his toe Jack nudged me lest I miss out on the fun. "Bruce says we could have made at least twice what we did when we sold the loft. Just by waiting six months."

"Really?" I rolled over, my head propped on my elbow and squinted up at him. "Then you could have doubled your contribution to the ACLU."

"Absolutely. We should have waited."

We both laughed and Jack reached over and patted Bruce on the shoulder. "Next time, if there's a next time, I'll give you a call. How's that? If I'm out of touch with such matters, it's only because with so many bright young robber barons like you around, there's little incentive for fellows like me to stay tuned."

A five-year-old with a tangle of red curls and china-blue eyes came to lie against Bruce's back, his small arms entwined around his neck.

"Your daddy's a pretty smart guy, do you know that?" Jack told him. The child grinned and ducked his face, not sure if this was serious or in fun. "And furthermore, he has a wicked backhand," and that made everybody happy.

We ate and schmoozed and watched the Frisbee fun. We listened to a discussion about the newly pronounced fatwa that invited the faithful sons of Islam to snuff out Salman Rushdie's life, as the proper price exacted for his having just published *The Satanic Verses*.

"But if Rushdie's agent hadn't called attention to the book before it went to press," said Jack, "I wonder if the Ayatollah would have given a damn. Or would, for that matter have bothered to read it. If in fact, he's even read it now."

Someone asked Jack if he'd read it.

"Only the first ten pages. Then I lost it. Or it lost me. Should I give it another try? But I doubt that I will. Nowadays I seem to read only what I enjoy. Deplorable, isn't it? But that's a privilege that comes with age, or at least with my age."

He was all of seventy-eight, and I thought of the books stacked high on his bedside table—biography, novels, whodunits, history, and always of course, whatever books came down the line about newspapers, their history, their objectives, their successes and failures. But as to the round-the-clock fare offered on television, excepting only the Yankees, the Giants, and the news, he had yet to be converted.

The sun was sliding over the sky's blue bowl and dipping below the tops of the oaks and maples. The midday warmth was seeping away.

"Shall we?" said Jack.

"Let's."

I rose and extended a hand to help him to his feet. Arm in arm we ambled out to our car.

"Here. Catch." Ordinarily he would drive but this time he tossed the keys across the roof of the car and slid into the passenger side. "You don't mind, do you?"

I backed carefully out of a tight squeeze and headed down the long, steep drive.

"So-o-o?" he asked in our time-honored shorthand.

"It was nice. Are you sorry we went?"

"No. Not really. How about you?"

"The same."

He reached over and removed my right hand from the wheel, placed it on his knee, and covered it with his hand.

"Do you know?" he asked.

"I know." And neither of us spoke the rest of the way home.

2

IMPRESSION: . . . On the short test of mental status today as compared to May, the probability that Mr. Stewart's memory impairment is due to a progressive dementing illness such as Alzheimer's disease seems lower now than in the past.

Dr. X

The next day by midmorning the sun was swaddled by a sullen sky. Gray-black storm clouds skittered along the horizon. The trees wailed and rocked, their leaves snatched up by a blustering wind. We woke a bit later than usual but there was nothing to urge us out of our contentment under the covers.

"Who goes first?"

"You. Tell me when you're out of the shower." I tugged the blankets higher and settled deeper, one eye on the darkening day.

A comforting sequence of sounds—the scrape of the shower door being opened, the rush of water, and then the door being slammed shut as Jack stepped in. Maybe I dozed because I next saw him, freshly shaved, already in his corduroy trousers and green plaid shirt. Standing four square before the bathroom mirror he slid the comb down his head, slicing in the part, and then with a few swift tugs of the brush he smoothed back his hair and tossed the comb and brush into the drawer. Even after all our years together, absurd as it was, I still took pleasure in watching him. It wasn't only his satisfying bulk, six foot two, solid, still slim, nor the high brow and square jaw, nor the black privet hedge eyebrows jutting out over the deepset blue-gray eyes, no. The quality I found most endearing was his absolute lack of self-awareness. Once a thousand years ago a flower vendor on Edinburgh's Prince Street looked up at him admiringly. She said as she handed me the roses with a grin that glinted gold, "Tis a baw-ny mon ye'ave thir." Not much had changed. In any land, to any eye he was exceptionally handsome, but had we lived in a house devoid of mirrors, he would not have cared and would in fact not have noticed. He was quite happy to sally forth, one black sock, one brown, his shirt, tie, and suit in riotous mismatch. He tied his tennis shoes with knotted laces and cheerfully pulled on sweaters with gaping holes for elbows. Until he quit smoking almost twenty years ago, he cheerfully wore jackets with holes burned through on the pockets thanks to his habit of thrusting a still-smoldering pipe into his pocket. On a winter morning, burrowing into the coat closet, he would emerge with anyone's scarf knotted around his neck. It could be mine, it could be one of the kids'. He'd shrug off my protests with "What's the difference?" and off he'd go, wheeling his bicycle out the door, his thoughts already turned to the work that awaited him on his desk at the *Times*.

Now tugging on a sweater he left our bedroom, calling Jeff to follow. It was a routine repeated without fail every morning since we'd moved full-time from the city to this house or, as we called it, "to the swamp." Flinging open the front door, Jeff prancing at his heels, Jack issued the familiar command: "Get the paper, Jeff. Go on. Get it!" And out he would bound, the coal-black, half Lab, half who-knows-what mutt, or "mixed breed" as the attendant at the pound so tactfully put it, and down the brick path Jeff would fly, his white paws hardly touching the ground. Impossible to watch without smiling as he rushed back, the *Times* in its blue plastic wrapping held high in his mouth, his white-tipped tail going a mile a minute. Jack had named him Thomas Jefferson, because, as he said, "We need more progressive thinkers around here."

By the time the coffee was brewing, the storm had erupted. Through the living room windows I could barely see the river. It was fading from view behind ever-thickening curtains of gray chiffon as the rain slanted in on a southeast wind. The marsh grass flattened and an incoming tide raised the water higher than usual out in the wetlands. A flight of Canada geese flew in from the river. As they crossed low over the house I glanced up and saw their white undersides, ghostly against the darkening sky. I waited and listened until their companionable squawking grew fainter and fainter and then was nothing but rain on the roof. Someplace I read that some American Indian tribes believed that geese wintered on the seas of the moon. I liked that idea.

We shared muffins and marmalade with the *Times*, working through the sections in our usual order: Jack with the front section. I with the Metro. Trade. He with the sports. I with the special section of the day, unless it was sports. Jack rated first go at the puzzle and both of us skimped on the Business section. Reading the paper I found it hard, no, actually impossible, to suppress eruptions of indignation or dismay. Invariably I found paragraphs, all or in part that positively had to be read aloud. A ferry, overloaded by 200 passengers, capsizes in India. No survivors. A newborn infant is rescued from a trash can, an eleven-year-old mother charged. Six children left unattended in a basement apartment, burned to death when a kerosene heater overturns. Starving refugees turned back at a border after a three-week trek on foot. Another attack in Central Park and an honor student, a piano virtuoso, or Holocaust survivor now hovers between life and death. Then, quite apart from the tragedies of the day, there was the King's English to defend: "Many thanks for the kind welcome accorded Hillary and I." Hadn't he gone to Yale, Georgetown, Oxford or Cambridge? Couldn't he at the very least keep his me's and I's straight? Jack, long since inured to my fever spikes of dismay, invariably managed a fine balancing act of agreeing in principle without tumbling over into outrage.

But this morning he left the table, hardly giving the paper more than a glance. The morning before we'd been biking for an hour or so and today his knee was bothering him. His arthritis was always worse a day or sometimes two days after he'd exercised. This had been the case for so many years that he hardly ever bothered to mention it. But a sure giveaway was the pronounced limp with which he walked.

All morning he worked at his desk, rereading a set of galleys sent to him a week ago. The book's publication date was hardly a month off, far too late to make any changes to the text. And in any case, the authors, a husband and wife, both of the Harvard faculty, had no interest in changes. Theirs was a theory that already, even before publication, was stirring up considerable opposition: *America in Black and White: One Nation Indivisible*. The book, so Jack said, posited that affirmative action actually harmed both blacks and whites. The authors further claimed that black people had made more rapid progression into the middle class before the advent of the civil rights movement or affirmative action. There were graphs and statistics to substantiate their argument. Although, as Jack pointed out, there was surely comparable statistical evidence that could be marshaled to prove just the contrary. Certainly theirs was a viewpoint that the average person would find hard to accept. The book had upset him. Since he habitually read many such sociological tracts, I was mildly surprised to see him so bothered by it. It seemed unlike him to let what was, after all, no more than an academic theory get under his skin.

I spent an hour or so at my own desk before drifting away from a humdrum assignment: a sidebar to update a travel piece on Scotland's western isles. The piece as submitted was fine. But, in a leave-no-stone-unturned frame of mind, the editor wanted to know what a traveler would find who journeyed to the isles in winter. Did the Cal Mac ferries still provide daily service? Were the inns still open? Restaurants? Were distillery tours year-round or summer only? All questions that would require a string of overseas phone calls to dredge up information that struck me as pointless. Information that once obtained, written up, and submitted would doubtless be deleted somewhere between my desk and the Sunday Travel section of the *Providence Journal*. I'd managed to put it off for an unconscionably long time. A few go-nowhere phone calls followed by a couple of busy signals and, sloth-like, I put it off yet again. Tomorrow I told myself, reaching for the Sunday paper and the puzzle not yet tackled.

Outside the rain continued unabated. Jeff disdained several invitations to step out into the downpour and instead curled up on the window seat beside me. It was his favorite lookout from which he could keep a watchful eye on the squirrels who lived, seemingly by the dozen, in the hollow trunk of a maple tree just a few feet from the house. This house, so fortuitously chosen, had turned out to be one of the wiser decisions of our marriage. Financial necessity dictated that we would both have to work in the city full-time and well into our so-called golden years. Jack's hours often, and mine occasionally, spilled over beyond the usual nine to five. Commuting, we agreed, was too difficult, too expensive, too exhausting. Our five children, three by my first marriage and two stepchildren, my "dividends" that came into my life with Jack, all were off and away, either married, at work, or in college. Living close to work Monday to Friday made good sense. A loft in a converted industrial building in a non-posh sector of the city suited us well. It enabled us to bike to our respective offices in no more than twenty minutes. It provided plenty of square feet for a non-stop flow of friends and family who found that bunking over in the Big Apple was an inviting option. Monday through Friday we relished Manhattan.

But come the spring, the urge to find weekend relief from asphalt and traffic, from streetlights that obscured starlight and water into which we could never venture sent us some fifty miles outside the city. Our house-hunting expedition culminated happily at a low, mostly-one-story house at the dead end of an unpaved road with only wetlands and the river beyond. We spent all our weekends there, confining renovations to nothing more than knocking down interior walls and adding sliding glass doors and wide, wide windows. Where a plot of corn had grown along a blank south side of the house we built a deck. From there, without even stirring, we could watch wild ducks come in for carrier landings in our own small pond. We could keep an eye on the great blue heron, stalking the perimeter on toothpick legs. In midsummer we could lie in bed and hear the love call of frogs. We often awoke to the haunting call of geese flying the night skies, softly squawking as they passed overhead. It was a house where we were able to live intimately with infinite light. The sun rose over the river, off to the left of our bedroom windows. Lift your head before fully waking and there was the dawn sky flushed pink and gold. Another round of sleep. Look again and the sun would be gilding all the tassels of the marsh grass. "Invasive weed" and "aggressive monoculture" was how agricultural experts spoke of such marsh grass. *Phragmites australis.* But maybe those experts had never seen the early morning sun tangled in their feathery plumes turning all of the wetlands into a bejeweled landscape. For how, if they had, would they not have been moved by their fragile, golden loveliness, and thereafter chosen kinder words.

By the time we were up and about, the sun would be around in the southeast and I could scoop all the pillows from our bed and toss them out to air atop the old stone table on the deck. In the late afternoon the sun hovered above the roof of the shed, flooding the guest room and the small screened-in porch, and before it set, its horizontal light would angle off the river's surface, turning it into a reflecting mirror of splintered glass. Ours was no remote oasis, tucked away into a wilderness outback. Yet we lived in delicious privacy. We saw no other houses, heard no passing traffic. From our bedroom we could saunter out across the deck to our outdoor shower, clad only in a towel or not even. To stand in the velvety dark of a summer night, the steam of the shower drifting up into a skyful of stars, was a simple pleasure, wholly satisfying. When Jack's retirement from the *Times* forced our hand and obliged us to choose between two residences, one in the city, one in the swamp, we chose the swamp. No easy choice. For it was not without regret that we packed up our city dwelling. It meant closing the door once and for all on the easy pleasures of belonging in town as a resident rather than a sometime visitor.

In winter with a wood fire in the living room and an unimpeded view of the marsh crusted with ice, the wild swans forming flotillas out in the black of the river, it was tempting to imagine that nature was reflecting our own inner sense, if not of peace—too quiescent that word—at least of contentment, an almost-guilty feeling of mutual satisfaction, of a fullness that asked nothing, needed nothing.

As always, I filled in all the easy answers in the puzzle, the two- and three-letter words, working my way around to the hard ones. On this particular rainy morning my brain seemed to be working at half speed. Finally, quite stumped, I wandered back to where Jack was still seated at his desk, pen in hand as he made notes working his way through the galleys.

"I need help," I said.

"Hm-m-m?"

"What's 'of homo sapiens two from one'?"

"How many letters?"

"Eleven. So it's not 'twins.' It's something o, something o. That's all I have."

He looked up and pushed his reading glasses onto his forehead and counted with a tapping forefinger the letters of a word still unspoken.

"Wel-l, how about monozygotic. Does that work?"

It did.

"I've never even heard that word. It means twins?"

"Correct. But only identical twins. It's from the Greek. Zygote. Fertilized egg. Mono. One egg."

"So what would you call fraternal twins?" I was teasing.

"Dizygotes. Di for two and zygote, same thing. Greek egg."

I was dumbfounded. "I've never, ever heard you use either word."

Jack invested words, all words, with a kind of sanctity more commonly reserved for religious convictions. If, irked beyond my limited patience, I swore, more often than not tending toward the scatological, Jack would visibly wince. "The English language is so rich," he would begin, "there's really no need . . ." to which I invariably tossed back my defense that rested heavily on Chaucer. "What about him?" I would counter.

"That was then. This is now. And if you can forgive me, you're no Chaucer. It's no excuse whatsoever." It was not his only inconsistency. "You hardly ever correct the kids when they swear," I'd tell him. "Why is that?"

"Not so. And in any case, I just hate to hear you use that kind of language."

But rich as was his command of English, there were some expressions he never used, would never use and which, whenever he heard them, unfailingly exasperated him:

lifestyle
win-win
a learning experience
body language
networking
bonding (as between human beings)
impact (as a verb)
at this point in time
zeitgeist
freebie

And these were but a few.

"How come," I persisted, "I've never, ever heard you mention monoygotes, dizygotes? Never."

"I guess because you never gave birth to twins."

"Very funny. But really, I want to know. Where did you pick them up?"

He shrugged. "Probably something I read."

"Such as?"

He laughed. "Whenever I ask where you read something, you always object. If you never can remember where you read something, why should I?"

"It just seems so off your beaten track, that's all. Biology, Greek, monozygotic, dizygotic. Not exactly words someone like you would be apt to use, or even know."

"Don't we all carry around excess verbal baggage? Words we know but have no use for? Of course we do. You do too."

"Yes, but still . . ."

"But still what?"

"Nothing."

"Then how about giving me some peace so I can get through this damn thing."

I swatted him with the paper and went off to put on a raincoat and venture forth with a reluctant Jeff to inspect the tide from the bridge across the inlet.

Lunch was black bean soup and spinach salad, leisurely enjoyed in front of a fire that crackled from logs still damp from autumn rains.

"Did you finish those galleys?" I asked.

He shook his head.

"Well, there's no particular rush, is there?"

"I promised to do a review the first part of this week."

"That's no problem, is it? As fast as you read. You must be well past halfway, right?"

"I guess."

"So you can probably finish it up this afternoon and get the review done tomorrow."

He didn't reply.

I glanced up from the mesmerizing fire to give him a quick once-over.

"Are you all right?"

"Why do you ask?"

I shrugged. "I don't know. You sound sort of . . . nothing, I guess."

He rubbed his knee and eased his leg from a footstool to the floor. "I'm fine. Just a bit tired."

"It's the weather. When it rains like this, especially in the fall, it makes everyone lazy. Even Jeff. Look at him there, dead to the world, not even caring that those two squirrels are playing tag not fifteen feet from his nose." He lay stretched out full length on the rug and when I spoke his name, he thumped his tail without opening his eyes.

"So would you mind if I lie down for a while?"

"What a dumb question! Why should I mind? A nap is a great idea. I'll tidy this stuff up and come in and join you."

By the time I reached our room, Jack, fully dressed except for his shoes, was under the quilt, already half asleep. I climbed in beside him and moved over into the comforting warmth of his length. His hand found mine and tucked it with his under the pillow in a sweetly familiar gesture, as comforting as an embrace. One-fifteen by my watch as my eyelids fluttered closed.

I awoke at two. Jack was breathing in the easy rhythms of deep sleep. I slid out from under the quilt, taking special care not to wake him. The rest of the afternoon I worked quietly at my desk. Twice I peeked into the room to see Jack still sound asleep. I wasn't concerned. He often napped, though rarely for more than an hour. But in the dark afternoon, with the hypnotic sound of the rain on the roof and the sills, a long afternoon nap seemed like a natural response to the weather. In mid-afternoon I braved the elements, splashing through the puddles to empty the mailbox out at the roadside. A long-overdue check from a publisher for a book Jack had placed for an author he'd represented for many years. Two other publisher letters, also for Jack, doubtless turning down whatever manuscripts he'd submitted on behalf of other writers. The usual assortment of bills, ads, and inquiries as to whether we had thought about bequeathing our estates to one or another worthy institution.

I placed most of it on Jack's desk and settled down to read the few letters that were mine. As I finished, I spotted the Sunday puzzle on the floor. I picked it up and, as was so often the case when I would leave a puzzle and then return to it later, I was able to fill in a number of entries that had totally stumped me before lunch. I polished it off, taking childish pleasure in completing the very last squares: 116 down—blank Martin cognac in four letters. R-E-M-Y. I inked in the letters, thumbed through a couple of the articles, something on Dressing for Violence, a high-style feature on boots and belts, manic hair, green lipstick, and jewelry made from bicycle chains. The political articles were no more compelling. Outside it was already getting dark and I realized with a mildly guilty start that the week had started off with a day that was almost if not totally wasted.

Five twenty-five.

I turned on a few lamps and then went into our bedroom. He lay on his side, his back to me, the quilt bunched boa-like around his neck, all but concealing his head. The room was warm, too warm. Neither of us had thought to open a window. In the half light he looked perfectly natural, still cradled in a long and lazy afternoon nap. I moved to the far side of the bed and gently folded back the quilt. The gesture released a brief warmth, a not unpleasant amalgam of wool, shaving cream, laundered linen, and body fragrance—clean, nutty, and lovingly familiar.

I laid my hand on his face and spoke his name, softly lest he waken too abruptly from so deep a sleep. Just so, hundreds, maybe thousands of times had I wakened the children when, as infants they napped in midday. From the depths of sleep they had to rise slowly, like swimmers submerged, floating back up to consciousness. Too fast an ascent would eject them crying and disoriented, unwillingly returned to light and sound and unwelcome exertion.

He stirred but only slightly. His eyes remained closed. I moved to the dresser and turned on the light, forgoing the bedside lamp that would shine too brightly into his face.

I spoke his name again, stroked his face, and sat down on the edge of the bed, taking his hand in mine.

"Hey, where are you? Look at the clock. The sun is almost down."

His eyelids fluttered then opened wide. His eyes stared intently into an unseen distance. For an instant I felt his whole frame stiffen with a rigidity that bespoke something more than fear. And then abruptly he sat up, his face frozen into an expression of unmistakable urgency. His words poured out, a twisted tangle of sound that made no sense. "The book . . . it's still in pages . . . errors . . . deadline . . . tell them, no, it won't be in time . . ." On and on, a dammed-up torrent. Meaningless. Insistent.

At once I understood. A dream. Still lingering. Still gripping his mind with a pervasive strength that blotted out my presence, blotted out the light, the room, the moment.

I wrapped my arms around his neck and buried my face in the warmth of his shirt collar.

"Hey. Honey. Wake up. Wake up. It's me. It's you. We're right here. At home. You're fine. There's nothing wrong. Wake up." Nursery sounds. Soothing. But also compelling. By just such words I would nudge him into the here and now, easing him free and clear of sleep's entangling web.

I drew back. I reached across and switched on the bedside lamp. I took his face in my hands and looked directly into his eyes. They appeared unnaturally recessed, cupped in deep, dark hollows. His pupils seemed enormous, twin black marbles rimmed by blue-gray circles. He saw me and knew me. But still his words continued unabated and my reassurances floated above us, unheeded, maybe unheard.

I rose and went into the bathroom. I held a washcloth under running water. I squeezed it out and returned to the bed and wiped it, cool and damp, across his face. As with a child I continued to speak, softly, imparting encouragement, reassurance. But a separate self, standing aside and listening, instantly detected the fringe of fear that shaped my words. In the pit of my gut, something dark and sinister uncoiled, expanded, stretching upward to spew a bitter, metallic flavor into the back of my throat.

Gently, carefully, I tugged his legs over to the side of the bed. He sat up but with no awareness. Perhaps, I thought, once he gets into the bathroom, relieves himself, gets the blood circulating a bit . . . Was I thinking coherently? How much sense did it make to urge a 190-pound man to his feet who was evidently not fully awake? Still, I stood in front of him and taking both his hands in mine, I tried to get him to stand.

But his focus was elsewhere. His efforts to stand were feeble, half-hearted, his attention was riveted on something more compelling.

"Will you help? Can you call them? It's already so late. It's never going to work."

"Of course I'll help. Who do you want me to call? What is it that's not going to work?"

But my efforts to fit logical answers to his illogical discourse got us nowhere. He continued just as if I'd ignored his pleas.

And then it came to me. A stroke. Of course. No sooner had the thought struck me than I felt oddly energized. It was a term, specific and definable. Idiotically I took comfort from its very specificity. Strokes after all were commonplace, were they not? People recovered. Even completely. Rest. Therapy. Good care. All would yet be well.

I eased Jack back down onto the bed. I tucked the quilt over him. I kissed his cheek and promised I'd be right back. I was conscious of the need for haste, for medical care, swiftly rendered. Hadn't we read a zillion times over that permanent damage could be allayed, could be totally avoided, provided the patient was treated promptly?

A longtime friend of Jack's, one of his authors and once a vibrant presence on the political scene in Washington, was in the process of recovering from just such an episode. Not long ago we had visited him in his Georgetown residence. It was such a pleasant interlude. There in their paneled sitting room, we sat cozy and safe before a fire, Burke, his ever-elegant wife, Fran, Jack and I. The room was fragrant with the scent of applewood and bowls of paper-white narcissuses. The thin spring sunshine of a late afternoon streamed in through the polished glass windows. Over a glass of wine, we listened to how it had happened. We marveled at Burke's good fortune.

"Fran was supposed to leave for Swampscott the very next morning. But thank God she was still here. She called the ambulance, had me in the hospital within the hour. If she hadn't been here, I wouldn't be alive today." He lifted his glass in a gesture of loving appreciation to his wife, who smilingly brushed aside the tribute.

"You would have been fine," she said dismissively. "You're much too tough to let something as minor as a stroke carry you off." We all laughed and knew beyond a doubt that only her quick response had saved his life.

Well, Jack, too, was going to be listed with the fortunates. It was simply a matter of acting speedily, intelligently, summoning necessary aid, aligning the forces of intervention. From the kitchen telephone I made a covey of calls. Mark, our son, only five miles away: "I'm on my way," with no what's and why's. Our family doctor: "I'm here at the hospital. Bring him right over. I'll meet you in emergency." The local first aid squad, all volunteers, so please try not to have any emergency arise between nine and five because every single member of the squad had regular day jobs. But cleverly, we had timed our emergency to dovetail perfectly with their end-of-day schedules.

Within minutes the whirling lights of the ambulance were in our driveway. I flung open the front door in welcome. With help at hand, all would be well.

3

Q: John Horgan, in his book, The Undiscovered Mind, *claims we know next to nothing about the way the brain works. Would you agree?*

A: I agree with him 100 percent. It's one of the things that attracted me to neuroscience. I thought, "Here's a field where you can become an expert pretty quickly because nobody knows anything."

Interview with Dr. Benjamin Solomon Carson,
Professor of Neurosurgery, Johns Hopkins Hospital,
conducted by Claudia Dreifus, *New York Times*,
January 4, 2000, section F, p. 7

The next morning I stood in the hospital corridor. Second floor, just outside room 215. The bustling efficiency that surrounded me was turned up to Fast Forward. Nurses in white slacks and smocks hurried up and down the corridor, parting to pass me like a river swirling round a rock. Bells and buzzers and phones rang ceaselessly. Unintelligible words from pagers, radios, and television sets wove a thick rope of sound, coiling out somewhere just above my head, just out of reach. Alien smells of artificial flower fragrance, antiseptic, disinfectant, schoolroom floor wax and steam wafting from trolleys of tired food, swirled into a cloying, heavy mixture. It filled my head. It would stick in my hair and cling to my clothes like cigar smoke in a Japanese smoke-free hotel room. In some inexplicable shift, all dimensions and perspectives had swollen into a grotesque excess of sound, sight, and smell—too much. Even the floor was too slick, too shiny, inhumanly impervious.

I knew the man in front of me was straining to maintain a grip on his patience. His effort to place his words carefully and sensibly in front of me was all too obvious. I was, after all, the spouse. Of course I was worried. Well, more than worried. Bewildered. Frantic. It was natural. People in this situation, probably especially women, could easily tip over into hysteria, which would be an annoyance, not to mention time-consuming. That was to be avoided and he was treading carefully.

He carried a clipboard and the lights gleamed and glinted from the stethoscope slung around his neck. When did they stop wearing those things like Lionel Barrymore, like Marcus Welby, the ear pieces holding them around their collars? Had there been some turnaround in med schools that decreed that henceforward stethoscopes would be wrapped scarf-like around the neck?

He wore a nice tie, a leftover summer tie of light blue linen embroidered with red birds. Cardinals? Probably. A good touch, doubtless selected to offset the all-white, antiseptic look of the knee-length lab coat. He had a healthy headful of reddish-blond hair and a tan left over from a summer's worth of golf or maybe sailing or tennis. His features, early forties, were still boyish and his manner was that of a man snuggly wrapped in a mantle of confidence. He had strength aplenty and some to spare in order to cope not just with his patient but with his patient's wife.

We stood, he and I, outside Jack's room, locked in an exercise that both of us were struggling to bring to a satisfactory resolution.

He was trying to explain.

I was trying to understand.

But the elements at our disposal were dismayingly simple. I needed more than what he had to offer. He would like to offer more, but what could he do? He was only a physician, a highly qualified neurologist. He was only a human being.

"I just don't see how it could happen just like that. So suddenly. Yesterday he was fine." I was bleakly aware that I was repeating myself. Hadn't I said more or less exactly the same thing only a minute before?

"We see it all the time."

"Just out of the blue? With no prior warning."

"All the time."

"And you're sure it's not a stroke? I mean how can you really be so certain?"

"There's no neurological indication. No hemispheric damage."

"I thought Alzheimer's came on very gradually. Over years."

"Often it does. But in many cases, and your husband is one such case, it can come on in a single, sudden episode. Delusion, disorientation, loss of coordination."

We paused. He needed to move on, but he was not quite sure . . . was I satisfied? At least for now.

I wanted to move on as well. But where was the gangplank by which I could fumble my way back to familiar, reassuring solid ground.

"So now what? What should we do? Where do we go from here?"

His hand on my shoulder was gentle, intended to console but also to suggest that whatever lay ahead would be structured and tidy. Would be categorized. No, we are not rolling chaotically out of control down a steep precipice. We're in this together, said that hand. You're not defenseless, not all alone.

But of course I was. Or we were, Jack and I.

"We'll keep him here for the next several days to get him stabilized. He's still having psychotic episodes. But that's to be expected. In a day or so I want to have a therapist work with him to get the swelling down in that knee."

"When do you think he'll . . ."

"Be able to go home?" A smile that, like the hand, was designed to reassure. "Let's see how things go. But I would think by Thursday or Friday we can send him packing. And in the meantime, we don't want you getting exhausted. We're taking good care of him in here, so why don't you try to get as much rest as you can at home?"

He replaced the clipboard on the counter of the nurse's station and held out his hand. "Call me at any time. Any questions, problems, don't hesitate. If I'm not available . . ." and then something about other doctors in his group. Totally bewildered, I watched the youthful figure, draped in white, a good firm set to the shoulders, retreat down the hallway. And with him went serenity, safety, and certainty in all its guises.

4

If you walk into a neurologist or psychiatrist with a relative who has got memory problems and they diagnose it as Alzheimer's, 40 percent of the time that diagnosis is wrong. If you use this data for research purposes, it's not reliable. It's not accurate.

Dr. A. David Smith, lead researcher in Oxford University's OPTIMA project (Oxford Project to Investigate Memory and Aging), *Saturday Evening Post*, March/April 1999, p. 76

Jack was admitted to the hospital on a Monday night. Discharged on Friday noon. The in-between was an unrelieved nightmare. He was totally disoriented. He was in Rome. No, Paris. The bells . . . did I hear the church bells? These people, they were dangerous. Not to be trusted. Whose side was I on, he repeatedly asked me. Agitation led to exhaustion, exhaustion to even more agitation. Metal bars were placed on either side of his bed. Nourishment was nothing more than sips of broth, cautiously administered lest he choke. Even the simple task of holding a cup or a spoon was beyond him. He was sleepless by day and sleepless by night.

I stayed with him from early morning until after dark, tiptoeing away only when his eyes closed and I thought, or maybe just hoped, that sleep was at hand. But whatever demons that had taken up residence within his mind were nothing if not indefatigable. Sleep was a destination that remained forever on the horizon, a resting place to be sought but never attained.

He turned his head constantly. His unseeing gaze roamed restlessly from the window full of sky to the overhead fluorescent lights, to my face, investing nothing that he saw with meaning or understanding.

His words, when he spoke, were blurred, half-formed, and almost impossible to understand. Occasionally there would be a sentence or half a sentence, seeping up from long unvisited crannies of his mind.

He had spent his childhood in a small town on the Hudson River. But it had never been his wont to revisit his early years, even though they had been spent in the midst of a loving family: wise and caring parents, a much-admired older brother, and a younger sister to whom he was pleased to extend both advice and protection. Once when we chanced to be driving north through the general area, I persuaded him to take a minor detour in order to show me the house where he grew up. It was still standing on the corner, shaded by maples, a white, shingled, two-storied house, unaltered save for the addition of a sun porch on the back. It could have served exactly as is for the setting of Thornton Wilder's *Our Town*. It was a house that bespoke cherry pie on Washington's birthday, overflowing Thanksgiving dinners, bikes propped by the back door, shelves spilling over with well-thumbed books.

But never one to indulge in sentimentality, Jack's take on his boyhood home was matter of fact, mildly interested but not nostalgic. It was in fact, of more interest to me than it was to him. When I said as much, he laughed and agreed. "That's as it should be," he told me. "Isn't the female of the species the nest builder?"

But now, in this alien, agitated state, random shards of his earliest years floated to the surface of his mind—scenes, scents, impressions, illuminated as if by rolling summer lightning before fading too quickly into a nebulous void.

On the second night of his hospital stay, having remained at his bedside until some time after 8 P.M., I returned home and was reading in bed when, around midnight, the phone rang. It was the night-duty nurse on the second floor. Could I return to the hospital? Mr. Stewart was becoming increasingly restless. Perhaps I might be able to calm him, to reassure him. The concern in her voice was very real and for this I was truly grateful. Another woman, a fellow human being was sharing this nightmare with me. From her concern I took disproportionate comfort. We were allies, she and I. Together we would yet find the route back to order and sanity. We would, wouldn't we? I drove over, parked under a streetlight, and stepped into the silent street.

The double glass doors swung open at my approach. I hurried through, bypassed the too-slow elevator, and took the stairs two at a time. But upon arrival, whatever ill-conceived optimism I'd harbored, abruptly vanished. "Restraints" had been ordered. I entered the room to find both his wrists strapped by leather cuffs to the bed rails. The sight made me physically ill, and for an instant I thought I would actually throw up before I could find a basin over which to crouch. I advanced to the bedside and laid a hand on his forehead, murmuring totally ineffectual reassurances. But no soothing words or loving tone could penetrate to the dark recesses where he had taken refuge.

"Undo me!" he commanded, straining against the firmly locked straps. His eyes were abrim with an expression I'd never ever beheld—dark, fierce, furious.

"You're with them. You're one of them. Why won't you help me?" He was hidden behind a sagging mask, a mask that had somehow come loose from its underpinnings. His face no longer fit properly on its bones. It was full of unfamiliar hollows around his eyes, below his cheekbones, under his mouth. Unrelieved exhaustion had leached his features of their natural color, leaving a grayish-white sickly pallor. His voice was rasping, hoarse, and filled with anguish. The sight of this tall, strong, handsome man lying so helpless in that bed, fettered and immobile, was almost, but not quite, as distressing to the night nurse as it was to me.

A restraint order in a hospital is not taken lightly. It must be requested by a nurse, and approved by the head of nursing. The request is then submitted to the physician directly responsible for the patient and, if approved, submitted again to the chief of staff. Once in place, it can only be removed by yet another succession of orders.

"It's nothing we ever like to see," she explained at the nurses' station. "We never request it unless we feel that there is a real chance of the patient seriously harming himself. In his present state of mind, Mr. Stewart's coordination is impaired. He wants to get up but we're afraid of his falling and were that to happen, we could be faced with a broken hip, arm . . ." Her voice trailed off and we gazed at each other in mute distress.

"If he could only get some rest," I began. "He's so exhausted, I'm sure it's contributing to his muddled thinking. Can't he be given some kind of a sedative so he could get a few hours sleep?"

Evidently not.

*

Midmorning on Wednesday I was privy to a diagnostic session conducted by the neurologist. It took less than five minutes.

Clean-shaven, neatly combed, this time sporting a cheery, canary-yellow tie with blue whales a'breaching, the neurologist approached the bedside, speaking with exaggerated clarity.

"Good morning, Mr. Stewart. I'm Dr. X. Do you remember me? We spoke the night you were admitted."

Jack's eyes moved uncomprehendingly across his face.

"Do you remember?"

"No. Who are you? Are you one of them? Tell them to let me go."

"Why don't you relax and let's just see if you can answer a few questions. Hm-m-m? Will that be alright?"

No reply, only unrelieved suspicion.

"Who is the president of the United States?"

To my astonishment, the question elicited a prompt, clear, and correct response, and I felt the first tiniest twinge of hope.

"Do you know where you are?"

"We're in Paris. Why do you ask me? Can't you see we're in Paris?"

"What year is this?"

"1946? No! Wait! It must be 1970 or 1972?" His eyes searched the face above him for some kind of reassurance.

"What month is this?"

Jack's eyes found mine. Telepathically I sent the answer. October. October. October.

But there was no one there to receive.

"Do you know your address?"

I held my breath and then, after a long pause, came a perfectly correct reply.

"Please repeat after me: 6 - 4 - 7 - 2"

Silence.

"Please repeat: 6 - 4 - 7 - 2"

"Seven . . ." Then nothing.

His eyes closed.

"I'm going to say a word. I'd like you to give me a companion word. If I say 'dog,' you might say 'cat.' Do you understand?"

But his eyes remained closed, though it was clear from the tense expression on his face that he was tempest-tossed and far adrift from the peaceful shores of sleep.

"Table . . . ?"

Nothing.

"Boy . . . ?"

Nothing.

Dr. X waited for one long moment before straightening up to return to the corridor. I hurried after him and my despair must have been all too evident in my face.

He shot a quick glance at his wristwatch and cleared his throat before beginning.

"When Alzheimer's sets in this way, when the onset is couched in a severe delusionary, psychotic episode, it's not at all unusual to see this degree of incapacity. I think once he's home, in familiar surroundings, we'll see a gradual improvement. These things take time."

Desperately I plunged off in another direction.

"You say Alzheimer's. Can you really be so certain? Wouldn't an MRI or a CAT scan be a good idea? And as to his delusions, isn't it possible that's he's simply light-headed just from exhaustion? He hasn't slept, really slept since . . ." I tried to grope back through a dark eternity to that rainy Monday afternoon. Was it really only two days ago? "If he could just get a good night's sleep. You heard him. He knew who the president was. He knew our address. He's just under so much stress right now. Strapped down, sleepless, not really eating anything. Can't you just change whatever he's getting? What about Prozac? Valium? Aren't they supposed to relieve stress?"

Clearly the chocks were out from under my wheels and I was rolling, gravity fed, down an ever-steeper incline.

What was the difference between an MRI and a CAT scan? I'm not sure. What did I know about Prozac or Valium? Nothing. Both were simply words. Both popped up with dependable frequency in print. Both were tossed around on occasion in broadcasts and sometimes figured prominently in books penned by authors who had experienced an epiphany, either good or bad, because of their use. My own personal experience in the pharmacological world didn't extend much beyond aspirin and toothpaste. And how often have we heard that there is nothing more off-putting to the high priests of the medical world than a layperson—me—trying to diagnose, much less prescribe, on behalf of a patient? But this high priest was prepared to cope with anything, including even a distraught spouse, one who was at a total loss as to how to proceed.

"We have him on a low dosage of Rispesdol. So let's wait and see. Keep in touch, won't you. These cases develop so erratically. We'll just have to be patient and see how he manages."

My expression must have telegraphed the absolute blank that was my mind for he quickly added, "Why don't you stop by social services on the ground floor. They can often be very helpful in cases like this."

One final smile and he was gone.

5

Alzheimer's disease was first described by Dr. Alois Alzheimer in 1906. Using a microscope to study brain tissue from autopsies, Dr. Alzheimer observed the pathological changes that he said resembled tangles and plaques. In the years since Dr. Alzheimer's discovery, progress in understanding the disease has been slow but steady.

www.mayo health.org/mayo/9903/htm/alzheime.htm

The question I'm asked most frequently, the question I most frequently ask myself, is, Were there really no advance warnings? But how do we define an "advance warning"?

Alzheimer's falls into that category of diseases and disorders characterized by insidious onset. There is no very first sneeze, no encounter with a rusty nail, no misstep at the icy curb. Alzheimer's denies its victim the solace of the pinpointed moment. And yet we're compelled to seek the specific incident, the sneeze, the scratch, the fall, driven by the illusion of control over the happenstance of life. In this compulsion to identify just such an exact moment, an undeniable advance warning, I was no exception.

Recently a friend and I walked along West Fifty-fifth Street in Manhattan, headed for a restaurant. As we walked she regaled me with an utterly absurd story about an ill-fated trip in Asia that involved a drunken tour guide, a broken-down bus, and luggage that flew off the roof of the bus into the weeds and wilds of eastern Mongolia. I carried in my hand two stamped, ready-to-mail letters and my car keys. We passed a mailbox and I made a hurried stop, just long enough to drop the keys in the box while retaining a firm hold on the letters. An advance warning?

What about that time that Jack and I spent in Tourettes-sur-Loup, a walled jewel of a town in the south of France, but a happy northern remove from the bumper-to-bumper Côte d'Azur. For two days we wandered its crookedy streets, and conversed with the artisans who had taken profitable refuge within its walls. We watched weavers and puppet-makers at work. It was March, too early for Easter visitors, too late for the cold, damp winds that funnel down the steep, stony gorge of the Loup river. We were in no hurry and nor were the residents. There was time to listen to the sunlit tales of May when violets carpet the hillsides. From the fragrant harvest comes a local liqueur called "marc," which we were urged to try, and in so doing were fully persuaded of its elysian properties. We shared huge square pans of pastry, topped with a smoky Gruyère and essence of tomatoes. Jack happily played chess in a noisy café with a cobbler who spoke no more English than Jack spoke French.

But that night I was ill and still ill in the morning when we were scheduled to drive a hundred miles west. Half the morning I remained curled up in the oversized four-poster while Jack packed, paid the tab, and loaded the car. Only at the final moment did I shove back the duvet, fumble into my clothes, and make my way to the car where I was content to do nothing more than doze and cast an occasional glance at our Michelin map, number 245. It was only after we were cozily installed in our host's farmhouse did I discover that I had left my all-essential notebook in the room where we had stayed, probably, on thinking back, in the bedding, doubtless buried under the duvet. A flurry of phone calls to the concierge and yes, "Voilà, le carnet de Madame. Nous l'avons trouvé ce matin, dans le lit." Which prompted Jack, despite my feeble protests, to climb back into the car, drive 100 miles, retrieve the damn thing, and drive 100 miles back to where I waited, sipping tea and spooning up yogurt in compliance with the strict medicinal instructions of our host. Was that my advance warning?

I've left passports in foreign post offices, countless raincoats on overhead train shelves, sent off unsigned checks carefully stapled to monthly bills. I've left umbrellas in taxis, books on subways, uncounted tennis racquets by courtsides, and let's not even consider sunglasses, gloves, and scarves.

When does ordinary (maybe slovenly?) behavior translate into "advance warnings"?

So if I apply my own scale of latitude to Jack, when and where should I cross a designating line by which the ordinary is separated from the aberrant?

It was May of the year in which the terrible diagnosis was pronounced. We had spent the weekend in Gloucester, Massachusetts. In the pristine Cape Ann Historical Museum we'd dawdled admiringly in front of the maritime paintings of Fitz Hugh Lane and Winslow Homer. We'd read and reread the incredible survival tales of men shipwrecked in arctic seas and listened in awe to commonplace accounts of heroism by ordinary folk who sought nothing more than to make a living hauling fish from the sea.

Over platters of steamers and jumbo lobsters, we met old friends and made a few new ones and tapped our feet in time to the sea chanteys belted out for the entertainment of our small group. It was a thoroughly pleasant, thoroughly relaxed weekend. We departed early Sunday morning. Why were we leaving so early? I have no idea. Probably we had plans to do something at home at midday or maybe early afternoon. Before the sun was even over the horizon we were on the road. As always we planned to split the driving. I took the first stint. The newborn green of a New England spring was on the land. Rolling south on I-95, a deep sense of contentment held us both in its easy grasp. Very little traffic, a good road. While the whole world was abed, we rolled on through the salty fringes of rocky Massachusetts, on down into Connecticut, smug and prosperous. Aaron Copland's *Appalachian Spring* was pouring in from radioland, the perfect accompaniment for this Sunday morning excursion.

About nine o'clock pangs of hunger finally worked through all that fish chowder, those broiled lobsters and steamers around which we'd wrapped ourselves all weekend.

How often had we both declared, upon rising from yet another groaning board, "I'll never ever eat again!" But now with the sun sliding above the treetops, we mounted a watch for a breakfast stop and found just what the doctor ordered a bit south of New London.

We took our time. As always Jack helped himself to a newspaper from each of several vending machines at the entrance to the diner.

"They all have the same news," I remarked. "Why get three when one would do? Not to mention that the *Times* will be lying on our doorstep when we get home." It was so typically me.

"How about pancakes and sausage?" he replied. So typically him.

We lingered lazily over a second cup of coffee and more editorials than anyone could possibly assimilate, or perhaps just more than I could possibly assimilate, before ambling back to the car. It was time to switch. I slid into the passenger seat and tipped the seat back. The sun full on my face felt fine. My last words as I closed my eyes: "I'll trade back with you on the other side of New Haven, okay?"

"Good," and he shoved the seat back all the way, folded in his long legs, adjusted the rear view mirrors, and eased back onto the southbound lane of I-95.

The next thing I knew my ears were all but bursting with an explosive noise, followed at once by a horrifying, metallic sound—loud, rasping, and terrifying. Smoke, steam, and a hellish smell of hot metal, oil, and something unbearably acrid was all around me.

The car was still hurtling forward, shuddering and bucking like some mortally wounded, metal monster. Bolting upright, I watched, as if in slow motion, the hood of the car wrinkle up like tissue paper and then all in a micro-moment, fold itself back across the windshield, blocking the world from view. We ground to a halt. I could hear my own heart pounding against my bones.

Jack's hand was like a vise on my arm. "Are you all right? Are you?"

Idiotically I nodded, as if the gesture were audible.

We hastily fumbled out of the seat belts, out of the car, and there, miraculously, marvelously we were face to face with assistance—efficient, courteous, and consoling.

"We were right behind you," said, according to his badge, Sgt. O'Dwyer of the Connecticut State Police. "We saw the car drifting to the left, into the fast lane, even though it was losing speed."

At fifty miles an hour the car's front left fender had scraped along a hundred yards of the metal retaining barrier. Had it not been for the barrier, we would have hurtled off a twenty-foot embankment with consequences neither of us wished to consider.

How? Why? It seemed all too obvious that Jack had dozed off, perhaps for only a few seconds, but just long enough to drift across the three southbound lanes until the barrier had held back the car's impetus, twisting and wrenching the whole front end of the car into a smoking, fumey jumble.

We leaned against the barrier, Jack and I, each inspecting the other for possible injury, all the while assuring the sergeant and his partner, Patrolman Lupino, that there was no need, no need at all to call an ambulance. We were fine. Weren't we fine?

Within an hour, the world was restored to order and sanity. The car was duly attached to a tow truck and hauled off to some unknown garage. The two of us were deposited at the New London railroad station where, in short order, a train would speed us to a station conveniently close to home.

Advance warning?

On an August morning we drove into New York. I had some work to do in the Fifth Avenue library and Jack had a lunch appointment at the Harvard Club, after which he planned to work on the club's September bulletin. It was published monthly, excepting only July and August. The first issue after the summer always seemed more time-consuming in its preparation than the other issues.

I generally used a parking lot on West Forty-second Street, between Eighth and Ninth avenues. Jean-Paul, the owner of the lot, was Haitian, and we always exchanged a few words about the dismal state of affairs in his homeland. Our conversation, from one visit to another, varied hardly at all. Developments in Haiti could be counted on to be *affreux, un désastre, épouvantables, tellement tristes, incroyables*—a rich assortment of no-nonsense negatives.

Our little ritual completed, I shoved the parking receipt into my pocket, and arm in arm Jack and I made our leisurely way east along Forty-second. The perfect day to come to the city, we agreed. Clear skies, hot but nicely tempered by a light breeze, low humidity, the kind of day when New York gives off its own special brand of energy that reminds you yet again how great it is to live on the doorstep of such a city.

We planned to meet back at the parking lot at four o'clock. We parted in front of the Harvard Club on West Forty-fourth Street. I paused to watch Jack disappear through the double doors, thinking how well he looked, suntanned, cheerful, looking forward to his lunch engagement, and not minding too much the afternoon's worth of desk work that awaited him.

I was back at the car a few minutes ahead of time. No problem, I told Jean-Paul. I'll wait in the car over in the far corner so as not to impede departing customers. I edged the car to the front of the lot, cut the engine and settled in with the morning newspaper. At four-fifteen I began looking up every minute or so, scanning the pedestrians approaching from the east. Four-thirty and I laid the paper aside, mounting a more vigilant watch. Four-forty and I was weighing the pros and cons of driving the few blocks to the Harvard club. But what if Jack should turn up and find no car, no me? Why hadn't I handed the parking receipt to Jack so he would have the exact address? But the answer to that was easy enough: he was even more apt to lose it than I was. But at the very least, I should have copied down the exact address. But what if he had had an accident? Such things happen. A mugging? Crossing a street? A careless taxi driver? Once your mind starts down that perilous path, there's no turning back.

Four forty-five. At five the club's office staff would depart and the offices where Jack worked would be closed and locked.

"S'il vous plaît, Jean-Paul, vous me permettez d'utilizer le téléphone? Un petit moment?"

In the tiny cramped hut that smelled of cigars and orange peels, I rang the administration offices, asked for Jack, and was immediately connected.

"Where are you?" I cried, fear and relief sending my voice into upper octaves.

"Where are you?" he countered.

"Where do you think I am? I'm right here at the car. In the parking lot. On West Forty-second. Did you forget? We agreed to meet here at four. It's almost five. What's the scoop?"

The voice that answered was not one with which I was familiar. Low, careful, and almost penitent.

"I went to find the lot. I looked for quite a while. I couldn't find it. So I came back here." Then he strengthened and found his customary assurance. "Wait right there and I'll be with you in ten minutes." But I caught him just as he was about to hang up.

"Don't budge," I said. "Stay put. I'll be in front of the club in no time." I drove the few blocks flooded with a relief so profound that it made my eyes sting. He was safe. We were safe. It was only a blip.

Advance warning?

And what about Jack's Thomas Edison joke, the joke that never failed to crack him up, the joke I sat through so many dozens of times? Was there a clue, even there, slyly tucked in between the guffaws of laughter? Was evidence of "insidious onset" to be found, camouflaged by absurdity? I clearly remembered the first time he failed to complete it.

We were having dinner with friends at some West Side hole-in-the-wall bistro, taking our time because, for once, we were ahead of schedule for an eight o'clock curtain. Four of us, replaying where we'd been a few days before when New York was visited by a mid-summer blackout. We were all happily bashing Con Edison, the utility company that all New Yorkers love to hate, which prompted Jack to head full speed into his Thomas Edison joke:

"Thomas Edison was hired by a great Indian chief to come out to the reservation where the tribe was having infertility problems." The groans that went up around the table deterred him not in the slightest.

"Thomas Edison looked the situation over and then gave the chief his solution. 'Oh Chief,' he said, 'You must choose three braves and three squaws. One brave and his squaw must spend the winter in a tent of bear hide. The second brave and squaw must spend the winter in a tent of deer hide. And the third brave and squaw must spend the winter in a tent of hippopotamus hide.'" More groans. But Jack, already shaking with only half-suppressed laughter, sailed on.

"One year later Thomas Edison returned to the reservation to check the results. He found the first pair of Indians had a fine papoose. The second pair of Indians also had a fine papoose. But the third pair of Indians had twins. 'Which only goes to prove,' said Thomas Edison . . ." and here, abruptly Jack stopped and poked me saying, "You tell them, Honey."

"But it's your joke. You tell them."

Which brought just the slightest flash of annoyance to his face. "Go on. Tell them."

I obliged. "Which only goes to prove that the squaw of the hip-popotamus is equal to the sum of the squaws of the other two hides." Which generated yet another chorus of groans, amiably mixed with laughter. It was his favorite joke. It played to his love of language, his delight in shuffling words the way a gambler shuffles cards. I was not keen about having to deliver his punch line but who would tarry over something so trivial?

But after that, I noticed, not at once, but maybe the second or third time it happened, when Jack would haul out his Thomas Edison old chestnut, deliver it with all of his usual relish, but come time for the punch line, he would turn to me, bidding me "Tell them!"

Each time the scenario unfolded I would feel a pang of annoyance and would resolve to speak up when we were next alone, asking him to knock it off. It wasn't funny anymore. But I don't recall that I ever followed up. Either I forgot, or if I remembered I dismissed the impulse as hardly worth even a minor dispute. But after that first Con Edison blackout evening, I don't believe I ever heard Jack complete his beloved joke, stymied evidently by the slightly tricky word sequence on which it depended.

6

An estimated 14 million baby boomers are living with a sentence of Alzheimer's disease today," [Dr. Steven] de Kosky said. He noted that baby boomers enter the age of highest risk in about 2020, when the oldest of them approach 75, and by 2030 the total number of Americans with the disease will double from current totals.

www.alz.org/news/right.htm, March 21, 2000

Jack, reinstated in his home, was a sad facsimile of his former self. He was unable to lift himself from a prone to a sitting position in his bed. He could manage the brief journey from bed to bathroom and back only with a walker and with watchful attention, lest he lose his balance, which remained considerably impaired. His appetite gradually returned, but the task of moving spoon or fork from tray to mouth was beyond him. The world swam before his eyes in a confusion of names and faces. His inner clock, his mental calendar, had been scrambled, and at first he had little or no energy for any mental reorganization. His days passed in long naps, brief journeys around the house on the walker, and quiet interludes when I would sit beside him, holding his hand as I recounted small snippets of family news, national scandals, and international upheavals. At times he heard me and replied coherently. But more often than not his attention waned within moments and fatigue won him over.

Before Jack's illness, I had traveled once or twice a week to the city, meeting editors, doing library research, completing the assignments that made up my freelance writing existence. Less than a career, more than a hobby, it produced a modest but welcome source of income. But now life had taken an abrupt and terrifying turn. It was unthinkable to do anything other than cancel all activities that did not pertain directly and totally to Jack and his care. It was not only what seemed most in his interest, it was also what I wanted. In fact, when I tried to direct my attention to an unfinished assignment, to a piece of business correspondence or even a long-delayed phone call in response to an inquiry, I found myself foundering. I was unable to focus. I couldn't remember pertinent dates, the names of sources. Deadlines floated past me. Always in the past I had prided myself on meeting such deadlines. Never had I had to plead for an extension, laying the blame on illness, computer breakdown, or the inaccessibility of an interviewee. But seemingly overnight that pride and urgency had evaporated. Everything but Jack was reduced to trivia.

It was a mind-set that seemed permanently in place. All day, every day was dedicated to the minuscule details that make up an invalid's care. A boiled egg for breakfast or oatmeal? How much water was he getting? Could a five-minute walk around the house be extended by a minute or two? Could he be persuaded to lift the one-pound weights a few more times in order to strengthen his shoulders and arms? Did he want to spend a few minutes with friends who stopped by or was the effort too much today? Could they come by tomorrow instead? Improvement came in almost imperceptible increments.

I had heard the expression "tunnel vision," but our day-to-day routine was best described as "tunnel existence." October folded into November, bringing with it all the preliminary hoopla that has come to typify the holidays. Jack was unaware of the calendar, and I, though all too aware of month and day, felt not the slightest inclination to partake of ritual or celebration.

Nonetheless, Jack was the much-beloved patriarch of our family. Our five children and twelve grandchildren were scattered across the country, some within easy driving distance, others on the West Coast. But even a continent's worth of distance had in no way loosened the loving bonds by which Jack was tied to the rest of the family. For the teenagers he had a gift for cutting through to the nub of complications that invariably arose in their young lives.

He himself, a child of the Great Depression, had started contributing to his family's household expenses at the age of fourteen. A summer job at a nearby school gave him dominion over the school tennis courts. Twice a day they had to be rolled, sprinkled, and swept. His minimal salary was supplemented by the privilege of playing on any court not in use. It was a deal he deemed more than fair. A couple of years later, looking for summer employment, Jack applied at a posh yacht club for the job of transporting boat owners to and from their boats, moored at buoys in the harbor. The job entailed running and maintaining a dory powered by an outboard. For all his diligence and dependability, he was not, to put it mildly, mechanically inclined. Could he manage the outboard?

he was asked in the job interview. A good question and one best not met head on.

"I grew up on the banks of the Hudson," was his honest answer and the job was his.

His was a boyhood that engendered a dim view of experiences intended to help the young "find themselves."

"Get a job," was his inevitable advice. "If you find something you like and if you're good at it, fine! It will give you a jump in helping you make up your mind what you want to do. If you're not good at it, if you hate it, well that's just as valuable. It's just as important to know what you don't want to do as it is to find your true calling." It was the kind of commonsense, no-frills advice that seemed in short supply among the so-called Gen-X'ers, the Me Generation, the Baby Boomers.

The younger children knew they were always assured a place on his lap for an animated reading of *Babar, Curious George*, or *Good-night Moon*. He delighted in teasing them and they in turn took delight in being teased.

"What's with you, Charlie?" Jack to a four-year-old.

"You know my name's not Charlie."

"You look like a Charlie to me."

"No, no," amidst uncontrollable giggles. "My name is Mariah" . . . or Owen or Eliza.

"Well, you look like a Charlie to me. So give me five."

And always of course there was his prowess on the tennis court that had even the college-age jocks in the family shaking their heads in rueful admiration. At the end of a match, on the last point, Jack delighted in swatting one last ball by swinging the racquet behind his back and connecting with one final pow-erful whack coming through between his knees. The coup de grace.

Because we lived less than a mile from the beach and the ocean, it was no surprise that as soon as warm weather rolled around, a parade of children and grandchildren made our house their head-quarters. There was always someone around to fill out a foursome for tennis. There were always enough bicycles lying around to supplement transportation to the beach. Summer nights were made for picnics at the beach or for lazy, late evening suppers out on the deck. Life was sweet in no small part because it was multigenerational.

So as Thanksgiving and Christmas approached, I was acutely aware that we had an obligation to the children and grandchildren not to spoil the holidays. Nor did I want the younger children to be alarmed by Jack's diminished condition. Sickness, infirmity, and old age can be distressing to a child. I was determined to do what I could to minimize that distress. By Thanksgiving, Jack was able to sit briefly at the table. Fully dressed, combed, brushed, and buffed to a gloss, he looked as handsome as in years gone by. It was interesting to note that he could summon reserves when others were around that were not in evidence when we were alone. Names largely escaped him, but he remembered faces, and for short periods of time he could hold up his end of conversations.

We begged off Thanksgiving dinner but were pleased to accept an invitation to join the family table for dessert. The day was being celebrated at Mark's house. His wife, Sarah, she of soft-spoken charm, was a cook of dazzling expertise. Dinner at Mark and Sarah's was a guarantee not just of lively conversation but also of memorable menus and a table graced with greenery and candle-light. Mariah and Rachel, ages three and five, bounced in and out of the celebration, free to come and go as they pleased and under no compulsion to "sit up and eat what's on your plate."

We were eight adults at table, and though we lingered less than an hour, Jack acquitted himself with honor. After coffee we pulled on coats and scarves and with Mark at his father's elbow, we made our way down the steps to the driveway. Folding Jack into the car, any car, was never easy. His legs were too long, his head was too high. But with Mark's strong arm and wise-cracking encouragement, it was managed without incident. I turned the key and headed off down the drive, braking just in the nick to allow a buck and a doe to dart across in front of us.

Jack's illness, devastating as it was, left him oddly incurious as to what had befallen him. A man of relentless intellectual curiosity, why, I wondered, had he never questioned me or anyone else about what was happening to him. But that night, as we drove home in the dark, he reached over and laid a hand on the back of my neck and asked, "How was I?"

Unable to speak around the sudden lump that filled my throat, I simply nodded.

*

Nowadays, looking at family photographs that were taken that Christmas, I could easily be persuaded that Jack was fine. It was unusually mild weather, so mild that the holiday gathering spilled out of doors onto the south-facing deck of our daughter and son-in-law's house, a two-hour drive from where we lived. Cathy and Stephen were determined to make it a festive day, and so it was. We were thirty-some strong, a group that included friends, neighbors, infants, toddlers, and all ages in between. Someone snapped a picture of Jack, flanked by his son, Mark, and his nephew, Terry. They stand, three handsome men, two in the healthy prime of life and Jack, unquestionably the senior of the trio, but a senior that gives no outward sign of infirmity. Mark and Terry are holding beers and Jack, glass in hand, is caught between sips of ginger ale. Only the most critical eye would note that he stands slightly more stooped. He gazes straight into the camera's lens, but his expression is devoid of ebullience, curiosity, protest, or laughter, although passivity was hardly a trait that anyone would ever have ascribed to him.

That day he walked cautiously, his sense of balance largely, though not completely, restored. A cane, when he could lay hands on it, was helpful, but the knack of keeping it with him did not come easily. His condition, his diagnosis, was known to all the adults present. They responded with words of praise, gentle encouragement, and the kind of good cheer that his presence at any family gathering had always engendered. But by late afternoon he was more than willing to retire to the guest room where, hardly had his head touched the pillow than he fell deeply asleep.

As the festivities wound down, we drifted indoors and by nightfall were grateful for the open fire. "So what are your plans?" I was asked, the question couched in loving concern.

"My plans?" I guess I had none.

"Have you thought of joining an Alzheimer's support group? There are such things, you know. Probably right in your immediate area."

I had to confess I hadn't. "I really don't have time," was my less than convincing answer.

"And what about your work? Are you going to give it all up?"

Good question. I hadn't really thought it through.

No one insisted. No one pressed me. One day at a time was my less than brilliant credo.

The following morning when we departed for home, Cathy, the eldest of our brood, walked with us to the car and in parting, folded her arms lovingly around me and laid her head on my shoulder. For a very long moment, we stood there, wordless, saying everything there was to say in that shared silence.

7

The ultimate goal of treatment and management of Alzheimer's disease is to reverse, reduce or retard the mental and behavioral process of dementia. Although headlines may tout the promise of new drugs to treat Alzheimer's disease, most such drugs are still in some stage of testing. And all, including the few currently available, are designed to treat some of the manifestations of the disease. None offers a cure of the underlying illness.

www.mayohealth.org/mayo/9804/htm/alztreat.htm

As a motto, "One day at a time" seemed about as useful as its alternatives, which is to say, not very. But in mid-January I was treated to a two-part wake-up call not easily ignored. The first part consisted of a long morning devoted to bills, upcoming taxes, a folderful of business correspondence, memos, calendar entries—all of which had always been strictly Jack's concern. Our finances were simple and so were our financial responsibilities. The coming-in and the going-out seemed always to be maintained in a kind of approximate parity. But that morning, wading through the paperwork, I discovered an alarming disequilibrium. We were in debt. My first, utterly absurd reaction, was a flush of relief that Jack would not know. But then, of course, came the more sober realization that staying afloat financially was going to be an ever-pressing issue.

I was fast making friends with the unexpected. But my definition of the unexpected was confined to what happened to others. Not to me. Then, suddenly, even that truism was shattered. One snowy morning, I awoke to find that I was unable to sit up, unable to turn over or even to stretch my legs out completely. The slightest movement caused excruciating back pain. The journey from bed to bath and back took thirty minutes or more and could only be accomplished in unrelieved agony. "Back spasms," announced our family doctor, the diagnosis pronounced by phone since there was no question of my being able to get from my bed to his examining room. I couldn't walk, much less drive.

"But why?" I wailed. "I haven't lifted anything heavy, haven't exerted myself in any weird fashion. What in the world could bring this on?"

"Stress."

"Stress?" I echoed in wonder. The word seemed too simple and wholly inadequate for the pain I was experiencing. His diagnosis duly pronounced, the doctor had little or nothing to add. Briskly he ordered up muscle relaxants, adding without too much conviction, "Try a heating pad. That might help."

"Is that all?" I asked incredulously.

"That's all."

"And how long will I be like this?"

"A day or two. Maybe several days. Maybe a week. There's no way to know."

It was a week. Seven full days of being unable to turn, sit up, or walk. Such abject helplessness infuriated and scared me in equal measure. Our household was not set up to tolerate two of us confined to the penalty box. One or the other, but not both. Neighbors helped. Baby sitters appeared, kindly women of incredible competence who ordinarily were only called in summertime when babies or small children were in residence.

It was a week devoted to graceless grousing, to total helplessness. But, in the long run, it was not a total waste. Just as an image on a developing negative floats gradually into visibility, two conclusions took shape in my mind with irrefutable clarity: first, any money I could earn would be exceedingly helpful, and second, it was incumbent upon me to stay as healthy and active as possible. For my own sake. For both our sakes.

Soon after slipping off the straitjacket of back spasms, I began rising before 6 A.M. Making sure that Jack was still sleeping soundly, I would head for the nearby YMCA and there within minutes would be slipping into the indoor pool.

*

Swimming laps confers a marvelous sense of solitude that frees the mind like nothing else. Once in the water, no one could speak to me and I could speak to no one. My ears were emptied of everything but the sounds of water, lapping, gurgling, splashing round my head. I glided along encased in a silvery tunnel of effervescence. Miraculously weightless, my physical self functioned in an effortless synchronization. One arm and then the other, drawing downward, trailed by bridal veils of glittering bubbles. Morning light, slanting in, refracted by the water, folded me into a cocoon of Monet blues and greens, endlessly wavering. One lap seamlessly followed on another, back and forth, back and forth in soothing monotony. My mind, unleashed, floated somewhere in the air above me, emptied, renewed, refreshed. One half hour. One half mile. My indulgence.

8

As the disease progresses, the person's exercise capacity will decrease. Helping a person with Alzheimer's stay as active as possible for as long as possible will help sustain their ability to perform self-care activities. . . . Exercise will also help make it possible to engage in purposeful activities. . . . This may help the person . . . have a sense of belonging.

www.mayohealth.org/mayo/0001/htm/alzexer.htm

Spring came that year with premature urgency. By mid-March willows drooped in tender yellow-green. From the winter-cold mud bottom of our pond, life stirred, ruffling the surface with microscopic life cycles. In the early morning the water would be dimpled all over by hatchlings. Walking in the woods it was easy to hear the turmoil of life stirring just below the top layers of last year's fallen leaves. Outside the kitchen windows the huge spruce tree was the residence of choice for finches, cardinals, woodpeckers, and raucous, squawking blue jays. It was, as always, the season of anticipation.

We took to walking slowly, carefully, down the lane, around the bend, and up as far as the small bridge that spanned the inlet to our pond. Where once it was Jack who would have pointed out the egrets, the herons, the swallows, that year, for the first time, our roles were reversed. Ten steps, maybe twenty, and then a pause. His hand on my shoulder was less a caress, more a searching for stability.

"Just a bit further," I'd urge him. "Let's see if the tide is coming in. Or flowing out. Last night I saw two horseshoe crabs, overturned. Stranded. I wonder if they're still there. Raccoons, even foxes . . . though what do they find to eat on a horseshoe crab?"

Ten more steps. Shoulders slumped. His hand tightening on my shoulder. The sound of his labored breathing not quite blotted out by the rusty call of gulls, hovering over the marsh, looking as always for an easy lunch.

In what month, on what day, did Jack's gait change so dramatically? Once, not so many years ago, we had a couple spend a week with us, old friends, both somewhat frail. H. was struggling to recover from massive surgery. Unsteady on his pins, he would gladly surrender to Jack, who undertook his twice-a-day walking therapy. Steadying him with one hand, his other arm around his waist, Jack would carefully steer him up and down the deck, endlessly encouraging and cheering him on.

"Heel first. Good, good! Put that heel down first. That's it. That's it! Step out. Heel first. Way to go."

Jack's effort to coax him from a slide-and-shuffle gait to a deliberate heel-first step was only fleetingly successful. Once released from Jack's tutelage, the gait of an invalid reasserted itself, as if even the sole of the foot was fearful of losing touch with terra firma so much as a millisecond. And so H. had replaced walking with the sad substitute of shuffling.

That spring, some time when I was not paying attention—but when was that?—Jack took to walking the same way, sliding a foot forward, unwilling or unable to lift it up and put it down. At his side, I imitated his very words of just a few years back.

"Heel down first. Heel first. Good. See! It's not so hard. Put that heel down, then step forward." And so he would. For three steps, maybe four. But then fatigue or loss of balance or coordination-breakdown would reassert itself and the steady, lifelong habit of stepping out, one firm step after another, would evaporate, and Jack would resort to walking exactly like our friend at whose side he had been such an indefatigable walking coach.

Our goal, our turnaround point, was the diminutive bridge, perhaps 300 yards from our front door. It was a legitimate place to pause. To take a few deep breaths. To debate whether the white sylph-like bird, tiptoeing through the shallows, was an egret or a white heron. And the ducks, streaking low, dark against the bright sky—canvasback? mallard? ring-necked? Peering down into the water, we would watch to see if the eel grass was being swept in or out, our landlubber method of determining the way of the tides. Always I would try to keep Jack distracted because the alternative was back to the house and his bed and the naps that were eating up more and more of his day. Turning around and heading home, I would be at pains to point out any small detail in the hope of turning his thoughts away from his own exertions.

"Look, off there under the trees, the wood anemones, not killed by that late frost after all."

"At least nothing discouraged the poison ivy over the winter. Doesn't it look bushier, taller than ever?"

"This afternoon at four they're going to show the finals of the big tournament in Palm Springs. Martina Hingis against some total unknown. Eighteen or nineteen. Unseeded. It should be pretty interesting, hm-m-m? Let's not miss it."

To all of these disparate efforts Jack, between breaths, would labor to respond. His speech, since his return from the hospital, had slowly improved. His powers of concentration were sharply limited but he was gradually regaining the ability to converse coherently.

"Palm Springs. Isn't that where we played croquet? At the opening of the Croquet Hall of Fame? Remember all that nonsense?"

"That was Palm Beach, Florida. This tournament is in Palm Springs, California."

"Of course. California. Not Florida. And who's playing?"

"Martina Hingis."

"Do I know her?"

"Sure you do. Remember, we saw her play just last September. At the U.S. Open."

"We did?"

"We did."

And wasn't it just as well, I thought, that the memory of that day had faded. Looking back, I could see that it should have been something of a red-flag warning that all was not well. But at the time, I viewed the day's excursion as nothing more than a long day that could easily have exhausted even a much younger person.

The bus, every seat occupied, departed the driveway of the tennis club around 8 A.M. headed for Flushing Meadows and the brand new, $254-million Arthur Ashe Stadium. By taking the bus and leaving the car at home, we would be avoiding not only traffic but also the hassle of finding a parking spot within reasonable distance of the complex. It was a cheerful ride with plenty of speculation as to the fortunes of the players scheduled for the day's slate. Jack was in good spirits, pleased once again to be attending the U.S. Open after a two-year absence due to nothing more significant than prior weekend engagements.

We were deposited just across the road from the stadium. The route to the stadium gates consisted of two flights of steep iron stairs and then a five-minute walk along a broad esplanade. By the time we reached our seats, Jack was visibly wilted and even though the temperature hovered in the seventy-five- to eighty-degree range, I blithely ascribed his fatigue to heat.

The women's finals was pitting Swiss-born Martina Hingis against the flamboyant Venus Williams, she of the amazonian build, the corn rows, and the serve that crossed the net only slightly faster than a torpedo. I wanted to visit the two adjacent stadiums where other matches were underway. Did Jack want to come along? He thought not. With his old white cotton hat to protect him from the sun and an animated conversation between himself and his pickup seatmate, he seemed in good shape, so I took off and was gone the better part of an hour. I returned with two sandwiches (outrageously priced) and a couple of lemonades to find him visibly distressed.

"Where were you?" he said accusingly.

"He was really worried," the man beside him informed me.

"I went to check on some of the other matches."

"You should have told me you were going." Censorious.

"I *did* tell you." We stared at each other, each of us trying to fumble through to some missing fact.

"I told you she'd be back, didn't I?" said Jack's seatmate, and instead of being grateful to him for trying to help, I felt only annoyance that he was sharing a moment I felt was strictly private, something that belonged exclusively to Jack and to me.

"Well I *am* back. And I brought lunch." I took my seat without a word of thanks to the Good Samaritan. Instead I stared down onto the center court, implying that I had thoughts for nothing other than the match being played there.

"So what's the score here?" I asked Jack, as if nothing untoward had happened between us. Did he recall that I had indeed explained where I was going? Did I think twice about why or how he could have forgotten? I can't answer either question today. Nor could I have found the answers that day. Peace restored, we ate our expensive sandwiches, careful to confine ourselves to incidental small talk.

Martina Hingis carried the day, winning love and four. Such an ordinary-sounding score that gave no hint of the incredible rallies, the impossible-to-reach shots that, miraculously, were returned, and with a touch so deft that gasps were heard all through the stadium. In the exuberance of the match, the confusion and dismay we had both experienced was set aside, not quite forgotten, but never alluded to again.

*

Suddenly a man who all his life had been active out-of-doors was confronted with serious coordination impairment. How now to find a way to let him continue to enjoy the outdoors? Yes, he could walk, albeit slowly and not without a steadying hand. Pretty confining.

Biking? Jack had bicycled all his life, and had biked from our downtown loft to his office on West Forty-third Street for more than twenty years. His idea of a lazy autumn afternoon was to roll up and down the quiet roads around our house with Jeff running in paroxysms of delight beside him. It was his favorite method of keeping tabs on the neighborhood. Two new German shepherd puppies at the yellow house just beyond the corner. The For Sale sign removed at the Tudor house that had stood unsold for almost four years. A huge dredge newly anchored in Polly's Pond. A family with four small children moving into the old Wilkins house.

Not only did he know all there was to know about the neighborhood, thanks to his biking forays, but the neighborhood knew a lot about him. He was by nature an investigator, a chronicler of events which meant that he liked nothing better than to pause to exchange views with joggers, strollers, dog walkers, baby buggy pushers, skate-boarding kids, and of course with the mailman, with whom he kept up a regular exchange of information.

Now all that had to change. A single unexpected wobble of the bicycle wheel could send him crashing onto the road. A broken collarbone, a concussion, an injury of any kind could land him back in the hospital with all the attendant complications of delusions and hallucinations. Subterfuge, duplicity and outright lies were my unappealing options. His bike remained in the shed, its wheels firmly locked with chain and padlock.

"A good day for a bike ride," Jack would remark on a fine spring morning.

"Which reminds me," I'd tell him, "we have to get those tires changed. Both are flat as pancakes." Flat tires one day, broken brake cable another day, and so it went until the day came when the bike was forgotten and I no longer had to pile one white, or not so white, lie atop another.

Tennis? Out of the question.

Swimming? Summer was fast approaching and only a scant mile from our front door was the ocean as well as an Olympic-size salt-water pool. "Oh, wait until summer," friends told me. "Even if he doesn't swim, just walking in the pool will be great for him."

And I wanted to believe them. But it was with something akin to relief that even that possibility nose-dived the first warm day on which we ventured to the pool.

I walked backward down the four steps into the pool. I held out my hands to Jack who took them and then stepped carefully down onto the first step.

"Great!" I told him. "See, it's not really cold at all." He paused and I waited, letting him grow accustomed to the sensation of the water around his feet. As we stood there, hand in hand, he let his gaze sweep over the scene, the long expanse of blue-green water, sparkling in the sunlight. The handful of people, sunning themselves, reading, in no hurry to share the pool with us. It was a totally familiar landscape, impressed into memory by more than two decades of summertime pleasure. But the expression on Jack's face was one of puzzlement as if he were trying to recall just exactly where he was.

"Take just one more step," I said softly and he did. Then he stood, one step above me, and looked full into my eyes with total lucidity.

"I can't do this," he said and I knew with absolute conviction that his words came from some perfectly functioning part of his brain, some segment totally unaffected by illness or degeneration. And I accepted his words without a scintilla of opposition.

"So what," I said, as we turned and departed the water. "It's not that great a swimming day anyway. Let's wait until the temperature gets up into the eighties." And that was the last time he ever ventured into the pool. Nor did I have many regrets, for who could say what short circuit might cut in when Jack was in the water, even if he ventured in no deeper than his waist? It didn't take much imagination to conjure up possible scenarios, all of which were like a cold hand around my heart.

9

In the course of monitoring the current medical literature, our staff at the Center for Current Research is occasionally struck by a project so promising that it should be shared with everyone. . . .

Summary: Studies in experimental animal models provide a convincing rationale for a role for estrogen replacement therapy (ERT) in the treatment and prevention of dementia. These studies establish the role of estrogen in the regeneration and preservation of neuronal elements within the Central Nervous System that are analogous to those regions of the brain most sensitive to the neurodegenerative changes associated with Alzheimer's Disease.

www.lifestages.com/health/alzheime.html

I continued to fret about how to coax Jack out-of-doors, beyond his simply resting on a chaise out on the deck. The boat seemed like such a perfect solution.

Our town was perched on a tongue of land jutting seaward between two rivers, both rivers emptying out into the bay. I never counted, but I would bet that where we lived, boats outnumbered cars. One driveway out of three harbored a boat and trailer rig. Half a dozen yacht clubs were active all year round. Kids in need of pocket money could count on finding summer jobs in any of a dozen marinas. Of course, there was the usual snobbery that placed sail over "stink pots," a point of view to which we were totally indifferent, for we neither owned nor aspired to own a boat of any kind. During all the years when we worked in the city and were in our house only Friday night to Monday morning, we found ourselves forever short of time. Two days only in which to do house repairs, cut the grass, bring in firewood, get to the beach or the tennis court, spend time with children and grandchildren, find an hour or two for bike riding. No matter how hard we tried, we invariably departed back to the city Monday morning saying, "We never got around to . . ."

Owning a boat, any boat, would only have royally compounded the problem. But now, with Jack unable to do all the things that he had so enjoyed, suddenly the idea of owning a boat struck me as nothing less than brilliant. I conjured up a dozen scenarios, each more pleasing than the last. It would have to be a powerboat. A sailboat would require too much getting up and down, shifting from one side to the other, loosening this line, securing that line. In a sailboat one has to move promptly and with dispatch. Definitely not for Jack. But a powerboat would be an entirely different kettle of fish. We would take sunset cruises, idling along on the river, watching the western skies catch fire. In the daze of the afterglow we would share a picnic supper and head back to our mooring as the moon lifted magically out of the sea. At midday we might anchor and I could dive in for a swim. Jack, of course, would have to stay put in the boat, probably snugged into a life preserver because, after all, you never know. Maybe I could take a book for reading aloud in a shady cove. Fishing? Well, I knew as much about fishing as I knew about boats, which is to say nothing whatsoever. Never mind. I had no trouble at all envisioning the delights of being out there on the river with Jack.

What a boot he would get out of my reeling in some finny delicacy—sea bass, bluefish, trout, whatever. He wouldn't have to do a thing. We'd head home and in no time the catch would be sizzling over charcoal. As we ate supper that night we would recall for one another the simple pleasures of having spent a couple of hours out on the river, under summer skies, far removed from disability and faltering prowess.

Somewhere between Jack's being stricken in October and the budding of spring, I had taken on, quite unawares, an objective that each day reasserted itself with ever-growing emphasis. I wanted to make him smile. For all of our life together it was he who had made me smile—his jokes, many of them so corny they could only be greeted with groans, his citing of life's absurdities, his unerring eye for the pompous, the pretentious, the overblown. It was the stuff by which our marriage was generously nourished. I missed his belly-deep laughter, his quick grin as he caught a conversational inanity that floated over every other head. Something had erased his spontaneity. Whenever I could orchestrate a situation that would make him smile, I felt a small flush of triumph, a wonderful sense of recapturing the essence of someone I was sorely missing.

Idiotic as it may sound, I envisioned The Boat as a way or rekindling for Jack some spark of delight. Once the idea lodged in my mind, nothing could have dissuaded me. It was reinforced even further by my finding a friend who harbored more or less the same fuzzy concepts of boat-owning. Doug was at least twenty years my junior, happily married to dark-haired, dark-eyed Sarah, who had plenty of other things on her mind apart from mucking around with boats. She was the author of several books, a self-taught specialist in Asian arts, and the capable mother of a young son and daughter. If Doug wanted to acquire a boat, fine! But count Sarah out. Her interests lay elsewhere. But just as I envisioned The Boat enhancing our restricted domestic scene, so did Doug visualize idyllic scenes with his kids out on the river. His son, once exposed to the indisputably wholesome fascination of rudders, anchors, lures, sinkers, reels, bumpers, painters, ship-to-shore paraphernalia, compasses, red-right-returning, and all the rest of the river lore, would surely complete the journey from childhood through adolescence in safety, undistracted by the sirens that make that journey so perilous. As for his daughter, well, maybe she wouldn't be quite so easily won over, but after all she would, in later life, surely cherish memories of long summer hours on the river, alone with her father, small interludes of sunshine, sky, and the luxury of his solitary company. Doug with his imaginings and I with mine were an ideal partnership. We would be able to split the costs of a mooring, insurance, and repairs. What could be simpler?

It only remained to find a boat at a price we could afford, one that would provide the minimal amenities we both deemed essential: a place for the children to get in out of the sun. Safe and comfortable seating. Ease of handling. Speed was of little consequence, and as for style, what did either of us know of that? So the search began.

Sometimes with Jack and often without him, I made the rounds of the boatyards and marinas, engrossed in the marine equivalent of tire-kicking. I must have been an easy mark for boat owners eager for a sale. If I was uncertain as to what we really wanted, I was on firmer ground when it came to what we didn't want, didn't need, and couldn't afford: frills and power and a megabucks price tag.

We finally settled on a Sea Raider, twenty-four feet in length, with an inboard-outboard motor. Built more than a few years ago, she was not exactly in the prime of life. But she'd had a complete engine overhaul, was in tiptop running condition, and furthermore was being sold by the owner of the local marina. We would keep the boat in his marina, right under his nose. Didn't that make great good sense in the event that she proved to be something less than what we were told? Done and done.

As if to prove the sincerity of my commitment, I attended a six-hour boating safety course, sponsored by the local Coast Guard and held in night sessions at our local public school. I found a spanking U.S. Navy hat at the thrift shop, and I spent several mornings and afternoons out on the river with Doug and a highly recommended Mr. Fixit who did maintenance work in the marina. Together we mastered the tricky business of entering and leaving the slip, how to come into a dock for gassing up, how to check the amps in the battery, how to read the channel markers—in short, how to operate the boat without life-threatening foul-ups.

I could hardly wait to share it all with Jack. It was a bright, warm day in mid-June when I drove him to the marina. Doug was waiting on the dock, ready to give me a hand helping Jack aboard. The boat was snugged to the dock, stern first. Climbing aboard meant stepping from the dock, over the stern rail, onto the seat, and then down onto the deck. It seemed simple enough. I gave a demonstration: "Just keep your hand here on this post and then put your left foot over the rail and onto the seat. Then bring your other foot over, like this. Step down onto the deck, and you're all set." But even with Doug's gentle encouragement, with his strong arm steadying Jack, his getting aboard was nothing short of an ordeal. Uncertain of his balance, unfamiliar with his surroundings, he hesitated before placing one foot over the stern rail. Then he waited. For an instant I thought he would step back onto the dock. Everything about his demeanor eloquently bespoke his reluctance for the exercise at hand. But gathering his courage, he brought his other foot over the rail and then stood there, too tall, nothing firm to hold onto, and only Doug's words and mine plus our outstretched hands to offer reassurance. But it was a reassurance that fell far short of what was needed. We finally had him safely settled on the port side, midpoint, his old battered straw hat on his head, his windbreaker zipped up to his chin. I sat with him while Doug played skipper.

The weather was flawless, The river never looked more sparkling, the water clear to a depth of two or three feet. The channel in and out of the marina was a cheerful two-way exchange of boats, moving at the required no-wake speed. Weekend salts (all of them a good deal saltier than us) hooted and waved as they passed. Bright pennants waved in the warm air and our engine was turning over with a silky-smooth purr.

I sat beside Jack, chattering away, pointing out details of Doug's navigational skills, exclaiming for the umpteenth time how different the landscape looked from the perspective of the water. A new house being built on a point of land, all quite unseen from the road. A boathouse once fallen into decay, now being rebuilt and even enlarged with a waterside deck. A big, grinning mutt of a dog on the stern of an anchored sailboat, diving and retrieving a small log over and over in a delirium of pleasure.

Doug never pushed the throttle past half-speed, careful not to have the boat leap ahead or turn too abruptly. But nothing that we saw, nothing that I said, made much impact on Jack, who sat rigidly, his hands braced palm down on each side of him. All of his concentration, which was clearly evident to even the most casual glance, was directed at his situation, with little or nothing left over to expend on the passing scene.

We passed the old boating club with its prewar clay tennis courts where once upon a time Jack had won the fifty-and-over men's singles. Remember? I urged him as we cruised slowly by, watching the players move like butterflies against the rust-red clay.

He nodded but his glance wandered restlessly away, searching the horizon as if on the lookout for approaching storms. Doug tried, too, but from the wheel he had to raise his voice above the noise of the motor and even then his words were scattered by the wind. And so our inaugural voyage, to which I had so looked forward, turned out to be a far remove from all my giddy imaginings. Jack was so clearly ill at ease. Furthermore, it was obvious he was making a heroic effort to appear to be enjoying it all, which in itself only burdened him further. Once when a sporty outboard carrying too many passengers, traveling at too high a speed, looped in toward us, veered away, and sent a high wake toward us broadside, we were momentarily pitched and tossed by the waves. For a split second I caught an expression of naked fear on Jack's face. It was enough to fill me with disdain for my lack of judgment, for my tunnel vision that had led me to believe that taking Jack on the boat would be a welcome distraction, a passive activity that he would enjoy.

We ventured out one or two more times with pretty much the same results. It was all too apparent that Jack was too distracted by the motion of the boat, by his fear of losing his balance, to enjoy the scenery, the river, the exhilaration of motion, or even the simple pleasures of sunlight and fresh air. Not once, on any of those excursions, did I ever see him smile. So much for The Boat.

10

The latest study, led by Dr. Ruth Mulnard, found no appreciable dif-
ference in mental functioning in women with mild to moderate
Alzheimer's who took estrogen in low doses, high doses or not at all for
one year. Some small studies previously suggested that estrogen therapy
might stimulate the growth of brain cells and protect them.

New York Times, February 23, 2000, Section A, p. 14

We all carry an inventory of indelible "historical shocks," moments
locked into permanent mental storage. Forever engraved on my
schoolgirl memory was that bleak Sunday afternoon in the hills of
Maryland when a voice interrupted a symphony broadcast to tell
of bombs falling on Pearl Harbor. A flawless June morning when
bells all over Philadelphia were tolling to call the populace into
churches and synagogues to pray for the success of D-Day. V-E day
amidst the apple blossoms of Virginia. V-J day, forever scented

with the pine woods of the Adirondacks. Where I was and with whom, these moments return with absolute clarity. I also recall, one by one, the trio of political assassinations by which the 1960s were ripped apart.

No less vivid are certain semantic milestones.

We were at lunch on a summer Sunday in the early 1980s. It was a bit more festive than usual because Leslie and Jacobus de Wet, parents of Marguerite, our daughter-in-law, were with us from Capetown. Jack, a longtime admirer of the writer Nadine Gordimer, was engrossed in what they had to say about life in South Africa, then in the death throes of apartheid. Nelson Mandela was still being held on Robbin Island, and the stop-and-go politics of his release were pushing all his supporters, among whom we counted ourselves, to the outer limits of exasperation. Conversation swirled amiably around the table until Jacobus, who was a physician, casually made mention of "sida."

The word brought us to a halt. Around the table expressions were blank.

"What is it?" we asked.

"A disease. Sexually transmitted. And invariably fatal." He held forth a bit on the speculation of its green monkey origins, supposedly in the depths of the Congo but we remained in the dark until our son, Billy, put us all straight.

"Over here," he told his father-in-law, "it's called AIDS."

But I heard "aids." Or maybe "aides." A word, not an acronym. Remember, this was the early 1980s.

"Acquired immune deficiency syndrome," Billy told us.

Just so, over a sun-dappled family lunch, did the world without AIDS come to an end.

I recall no such salient moment when, for the first time, the word *Alzheimer's* swam into my consciousness. But, like all the rest of us, I had no trouble whatsoever pinpointing its most prominent victim. Surely Alzheimer's and Ronald Reagan are forever linked in the nation's collective memory. But in the beginning Reagan's problems were not even identified as Alzheimer's. The Mayo Clinic preferred to call it "degenerative cognitive dementia." Even after his failing condition was duly acknowledged, he remained the Teflon president, seemingly unaffected. Pick up any paper and there he was, still slim, still erect, his shinola hair as black and shiny as Snow White's, his amiable features creased into a good-guy grin. He waves. He walks unassisted toward the camera. Who would ever guess that he was other than hale and hearty, as ready as ever to saddle up or chop wood for the next front page photo op. As my only available model, Ronald Reagan was really not much help as I struggled to make sense out of what was happening to Jack.

Speculation had long been rife as to the origin of Reagan's mental disintegration. Talk show hosts, members of the presidential staff, office interns, journalists, biographers, guests who graced the White House official guest list were all only too ready to go on record with their own views as to when and under what circumstances Reagan's first symptoms came to light.

It was hard not to compare the onset of Jack's troubles with those of Reagan's. Certainly, the now-famous letter that Reagan penned in his own hand on November 5, 1994, announcing his diagnosis, would have been well beyond Jack's capabilities once he was stricken. As a lifelong newspaperman, he typed his correspondence and rarely wrote in longhand. But now his attempts to type coherently were heartbreaking, and even when, on several occasions, he asked me to retype a letter for him, I was hard put to decipher what it was he was trying to convey.

Speculation about the presidential Alzheimer's could be had almost daily in the newspapers. I read much of it, but much of it escaped me. It was a longtime friend, herself a doctor, who mentioned, quite casually, the possibility that Reagan's illness was linked to his experience immediately after he was shot in March 1981.

"You know, at that time Reagan lost more than half his blood supply. He would have died within the hour had he not been given massive transfusions of whole blood. There's another consideration. Because of the dire emergency circumstances, the blood went into him several degrees below normal body temperature."

"And that could cause Alzheimer's? The low temperature of the blood or the blood itself?"

"Maybe both. Maybe neither. It's just a theory. Not proven but not disproven either. And anyway, no one speaks of the 'cause' of Alzheimer's. The truth is, we still know next to nothing about its cause. Its causes. And we know even less about how to intercede to prevent full-blown Alzheimer's. But it's pretty well an accepted fact that blood transfusions carry risk. You know that for a long time, far too long a time too, we didn't screen for the AIDS virus. Now of course we do. But what else is being transmitted that we don't even suspect? But then that's probably not news to you, is it?"

"No. Not really."

"And hasn't Jack had his share of emergency room transfusions?"

"I guess."

"So if you're looking for something to blame, you could start with that. Trauma. Blood transfusions." She shrugged. "It could be. And then again . . ."

"And then again what?"

She laughed. "You tell me."

*

From our loft on West Seventeenth Street it was only twenty-six blocks up to the office of the *Times* on West Forty-third Street. For Jack that translated into a bike ride of probably less than ten minutes, depending on traffic and weather. He had been riding his bike in Manhattan for too many years to be other than cautious. Indeed, a friend of his, also a journalist, riding his bike in Washington, D.C., had been killed when he slammed full tilt into a suddenly opened taxi door. I lost count of how many times he told me that story, repeating it as a cautionary note every time I wheeled my own bike out of our building.

On a flawless day in April 1990 he left Seventeenth Street, headed for his office at about 7:15 in the morning. Heading north on Sixth Avenue, the traffic was still light. But some time shortly after daybreak, city trucks had traveled the length of Sixth Avenue posting signs proclaiming Earth Day. In conjunction with its celebration, a bike lane was improvised by way of orange traffic cones placed at regular intervals of thirty feet or so.

In order to comply, Jack wheeled north, dutifully keeping in the designated lane. It happened between Twenty-first and Twenty-second streets. An oil spill. Was it heating oil? Diesel? Motor oil? It was never determined. The only detail on which there was no disagreement was that a large and messy spill of oil lay between the curb and the traffic cones, full in the middle of the bike lane. Headed north, into the early morning light, Jack saw the spill and mistook it for nothing more than a puddle of water. In less time than it takes to speak the words, his bike lost traction and spun sideways, and Jack was flung onto the street. He was knocked cold. His right leg was shattered from hip to knee.

*

Six hours earlier and six time zones to the east, in the southwest corner of France, I was setting out to explore Bordeaux, in the august company of Monsieur Jean-Jacques Jouet, director of the Bordeaux Tourist Office. Monsieur Jouet was tall, lean, and straight-as-a-pitch-pine. He was in his late sixties, maybe early seventies. In his navy-blue lapel he wore the tiny tricolor ribbon, the Legion of Honor. Monsieur Jouet was *un légionnaire*. With his headful of white hair, his matching moustache, and grave demeanor, he perfectly fulfilled my idea of a senior senator, an ambassador, a Nobel Peace Prize winner.

From his first words of introduction, standing in the doorway of my minuscule hotel, I understood exactly what had happened. Through some bureaucratic mix-up I had been mistaken by his office for someone else. Someone important. A television personality? A high-powered journalist whose conclusions could be heard on the nightly news? So instead of being consigned to some junior member of his staff, as would befit a freelance travel writer of my ilk, I was being escorted by the director himself. Not that he really minded, for the task of acquainting me or anyone else with the history and beauty of Bordeaux was so distinctly his pleasure. Bordeaux was more than just his city of birth. It was his pride, his pleasure, his *amour*. My good luck.

For three days prior to our meeting I had been touring the Bordelaise countryside from which come the world's finest wines. No need to hedge that statement with commentary about the wines from elsewhere. Not from Alsace, the Rhine, Australia, or California. Mention of any other wine-growing area elicited always the same reaction.

"Pouf!" and an expressive wave of the hand. Not ever to be compared with the glorious output of the Bordelaise vineyards. Three days of vineyard-visiting left me saturated with a dizzying array of facts and statistics—bottles per hectare, barrels per year, days or weeks in oaken casks.

Sip. Swish. Spit. Sauterne. Médoc. Pomerol. Pauillac. Marguax. Entre-Deux-Mers. Short in the mouth, long in the nose. The flavor was what? Oaky? Fruity? Smoky? Grassy? The trio of days was topped off by a visit to the impeccable wine museum at Château Mouton-Rothschild, steeped in an atmosphere so rarefied that one wondered how mere mortals were admitted. There I handled Greek flagons of clay, retrieved from the floor of the Aegean to which they had sunk two or was it three thousand years ago, and there my footprints along the white pebble paths were, within minutes, raked into oblivion by invisible caretakers.

At the end of three days I was saturated, satiated, and exhausted. I returned to center-city Bordeaux, despairing of ever turning it all into some kind of written form that would entice any readers, apart from hardened oenophiles, who doubtless knew it all anyway. In short, I was ready for Monsieur Jouet.

We hear often enough about people falling in love with Paris. But how often is there any mention of impassioned bonding with Bordeaux? I wonder why not. Seeing the city through the eyes of its lifelong admirer, listening to him hold forth on its glorious past, its auspicious future, I was easily persuaded.

In the late 1700s Bordeaux's bustling river port fit neatly into the lucrative trade triangle: Bordeaux–West Africa–the Antilles. A good fit with the New World's enthusiasm for slavery.

All that flawless spring day, Monsieur Jouet walked me through the centuries of his city. In the whispery gloom of St. Andrews Cathedral where, in 1152, Eleanor of Aquitaine married Henry

Plantagenet, he gently reminded me of the significance of that wedding.

"You'll recall, of course, that for the next three hundred years, all of western France, from Normandy south to the Pyrenees, with the sole exception of Brittany was ruled by England."

Well, I did indeed recall some such tie. But 300 years? No. As an American it was all I could do to grope my way back to Plymouth Rock, Jamestown, and the House of Burgesses. Indeed, that tumultuous period of English rule over fertile, prosperous western France was over and done with almost forty years before Columbus even headed west across the Atlantic. No wonder my countrymen are credited with such a short historical attention span!

In the shadow of the Great Bell, hanging high in the town's Gothic belfry, I waited as Monsieur Jouet checked his watch against the town clock. With a smile of satisfaction he extended his gold pocket watch for my inspection.

"In perfect agreement," he noted, snapping closed its gold cover and slipping it back into his waistcoat pocket.

In St. Michael's Church he pointed out an early sixteenth century sculpted group of children, and told me that the little girl with the winsome expression was the Virgin Mary. We sat in the sunshine before the Place de la Bourse. The early morning sun was casting a golden hue on the creamy limestone buildings. In elegance and symmetry the great open square was every bit as impressive as the Place de la Concorde and the traffic no less unnerving.

The Grand Théâtre was not yet open to the public, but a word from Monsieur Jouet and a uniformed custodian unlocked massive doors to admit us a full hour ahead of time. A majestic Roman temple of awesome proportions, it cost more than twice its original estimate and well worth every golden Louis. In the half gloom we mounted the splendid staircase and peered over the auditorium, a masterpiece of ramps, pillars, and cantilevered boxes. On stage a rehearsal of Molière's *Le Bourgeois Gentilhomme* was underway, the cast casually decked out in jeans and T-shirts. We sat for a few minutes to listen, and when I mentioned how clearly the dialogue could be heard, my shepherd told me that the wood used in the theater's interior was especially selected for its acoustical qualities. Both the Paris Opera House and Philadelphia's Academy of Music were in part copied from Bordeaux's magnificent theater.

After too much lunch in the Grand Balcon, we strolled the dappled shade of the Allées de Tourny and I heard how Bordeaux had fared during the Second World War. In 1940, with the Germans jackbooting their way into France, the French government moved its center of operations from Paris to Bordeaux. German bombers followed. Within a week bombs were raining down on Bordeaux. After one night's bombardment, the mayor strode forth to view the damage. What he beheld moved him to the brink of tears. Tears of rage. Turning to the newly arrived ministers, heedless of their rank he vented his wrath.

"Look what you've brought down on our beautiful city," he shouted. "Take your damned government and get the hell out of here." Meekly they complied. All was moved to Vichy and remained there until the war's end.

Monsieur Jouet told the story with energy, with animation, which I mistook for irony, not too far removed from humor.

I laughed and said, "What a great example of valuing aesthetics over essentials." And at once I understood how completely I had misread that small slice of history. Monsieur Jouet stopped. He turned to me, a perplexed expression on his face.

"But my dear Madame," he said, "Hasn't civilization taught us, no, not taught us, but commanded us, to place aesthetics above all else? Indeed, aesthetics *are* the essentials of life." And there I thought, in a nutshell, was the difference between his country and mine. Nor was I prepared to say, at the moment, which take, his or mine, was preferable.

*

It was early evening when I returned to my pint-sized hotel, hidden away on a side street, within sniffing distance of the roses that flourished in a city park. Monsieur Jouet and I took our leave of one another under the hotel's red and white sidewalk umbrellas. He told me what a pleasure it had been to spend the day in my company. I told him how much I appreciated his making his valuable time available to me. He wished me a safe trip home. I wished him a successful summer season. We smiled. We shook hands in a spirit of undoubted sincerity, undoubted cordiality. I pushed open the double glass doors and with a sigh, stepped into the welcome gloom of the minuscule lobby. It had been a long day, a day so filled with facts, impressions, and historical vignettes as to merit not an article or two but something encyclopedic in both length and depth. Something certainly well beyond anything I could hope to persuade any magazine or newspaper editor to buy. It was such a common problem that I had long since ceased to let it bother me. Inevitably, once I launched myself on a story in any area rich in history, I would find myself so immersed in the long-ago past as viewed from the here and now that optimum word lengths fell into obscurity. Always, there was so much to tell, so much to pass along in the vain hope that I could persuade a reader to match my own enthusiasms page for page.

I was almost safely into the birdcage elevator when a triumvirate of hotel personnel descended on me. Madame has an urgent telephone message from home. An accident. Your husband. A bicycle accident. Your sister, I believe . . . no, no, not your sister, your daughter . . . Jennifer? Yes, that's it. Your daughter. She will phone back. At nine o'clock Bordeaux time.

It was a breathless delivery, confusing but irrefutably ominous. Details were lacking but there was no mistaking the gravity of the text. Was there a number where Jennifer could be reached? Was there any suggestion of what hospital my husband was in? The nature of his injuries . . . had that been mentioned? Hèlas, no. Nothing specific. No details.

I could feel my heart skittering inside its rib cage. Scrambling for out. A dark, salty taste filled my mouth and my knees went wobbly. I hung on. Careful. Careful. Stay calm. Just listen.

The trio of faces in front of me, the patent-haired hotel owner, his gentle bosomy wife, and their pretty manager-daughter who was studying hotel management in Lyons, were all suffused with kindly concern. There would be a three-hour wait before Jenny would be calling. Was there anything Madame wished in the interval?

A time compressor. Something that would swallow up the three-hour interval. But apart from that, what could dispel the dread I was breathing in, thick as fog, dread to be tasted, even smelled, rank, primordial. No. Yes, thank you. Really, I'm fine. Most kind. Yes, of course I'll let you know. And the gates of the birdcage elevator closed and I rose, gazing down on the bald, the bunned, and the blonde-braided heads, all three tilted worriedly upward.

Today I suppose the fearsome time that followed would be totally avoidable. Who waits these days for something as simple as an overseas phone call? Beepers, pagers, cell phones, satellites, and microchips seem to have obliterated the distance once imposed by oceans, mountains, deserts, even outer space. But in those far-off days life moved at a different pace. From my room a call to the U.S. involved lifting the phone, requesting *une ligne à l'extérieure*, which often as not was unavailable. Would I please hang up and when such a line became available, I would be called. When or if I was finally called back and I requested the number in the U.S., it was not at all unusual to hear that all the circuits were busy. Please try your call later.

But where would I call anyway? I had no idea where Jack was. In a hospital, I presumed. But which one? And Jenny? Where was she? Doubtless with her father, but if she said she would call in three hours, I knew with a bone-deep certainty that she would. Furthermore, my inane efforts to place a call myself might very well obstruct her efforts to reach me. The tidy convenience of Call Waiting had yet to be born.

I tried to read, but the words floated off the page. Read aloud, I told myself. But that didn't work either. My voice sounded dry and cracked. Then tidy up your notes, those half-completed words hurriedly scribbled throughout the day in my small red spiral notebook. That helped, but in less than ten minutes the task seemed overwhelming. My mind was spiraling off, sucking in image after image, each more unbearable than the last. A head injury with loss of memory or speech? Or maybe spinal damage with paralysis, respirator, wheelchairs, ramps, and abject helplessness. Stop! *Stop!* Go for blank. Total blank. A high wall behind my eyelids, a vacuum, sealed tight and then, by habit, the reaching out for memorized poetry, long-ago lines, worn thin with use on all the nights when sleep hovered just out of reach.

Dim drums throbbing in the hills half heard. With rue my heart is laden. Such a good word, rue. Whatever happened to rue? By brooks too broad for leaping . . . Old Noah walking round his ark looked through the window pane. . . . Is the winter of our discontent made glorious summer? Home is the hunter, home from the hill. . . . And may there be no mourning. Was it mourning *or maybe* moaning? *When I set out to sea. . . . Left undone the things we ought to have done and something something and no health in us. . . . And the fish of the sea and whatsoever passeth through the paths of the sea. . . . So conceived and so dedicated can long endure. . . . Just plain Bill from over the hill. . . . But don't stop or the wall will crumble and reality will wash through as insistent as surf. Little Billy in one of his brand new sashes, fell in the fire, and was burned to ashes. Now it's getting rather chilly. . . .*

The phone jangled by my ear. I woke up. How could I possibly have slept? The treachery of sleep! Confusion and dread rushed in, liberally laced with guilt.

Pre-satellite, pre-coaxial cable, by whatever means that then prevailed, Jenny's voice came through, so sweetly familiar it brought tears to my eyes. I sat rigidly on the edge of the bed, pressing the telephone into my head with a mindless kind of force. As I listened I watched but scarcely saw the city come twinkling into life and heard but didn't hear far-off church bells tolling the hours, rolling out the sound in huge leaden balls above the rooftops.

11

Researchers have identified several nongenetic factors that may affect people's odds [for getting Alzheimer's disease]. Head injury is probably the best documented. Researchers know from autopsy studies that head trauma can cause an acute buildup of amyloid plaque, and epidemiological surveys suggest those sudden deposits can have long-term consequences. In a five-year study involving 2,000 elderly New Yorkers, Dr. Richard Mayeux of Columbia University found that those who'd been knocked unconscious as adults developed Alzheimer's at three times the rate of those who hadn't.

Geoffrey Cowley, *Newsweek*, January 31, 2000, p. 50

Haven't we all been told, not once, but over and over again, never to let ourselves be carried into the emergency ward of any big city hospital. Horror stories abound. The wounded, the terminally ill, sitting or lying in waiting rooms, unattended, ignored, the juice of life seeping away while chattering personnel hurry by discussing love lives, baseball scores, or recipes. We had a good friend from Philadelphia whose account of just such an experience we passed around, person to person, in awed and fearful tones. A misstep on a Manhattan curb of an early winter evening, a broken shoulder and dislocated arm, hideous pain, shock. Fortunate at least in successfully flagging a cab, into which he dropped, barely conscious, pleading to be taken to the nearest hospital. A lurching ride, a rude exchange over the fare, the tip, and then two hours on a plastic chair in an Upper East Side hospital while an attendant in a glass booth read the evening tabloid, only looking up long enough to tell the lame and the halt, "Have a seat. Someone will see you shortly." The rest of the story involved hailing yet another cab, another jolting interval until he was deposited on the doorstep of a downtown hospital. There his out-of-state insurance credentials were skeptically viewed. Only after he had signed a blank personal check that was then clipped to two major credit cards was he examined by a trainee, his clothes replaced with a hospital gown, and told that he was scheduled for X-ray, and probably surgery, "sometime tomorrow morning." After 24 god-awful hours, he managed to make his way back to Philadelphia, where, within the week, the surgery had to be repeated. A bill in the five figures pursued him for the better part of a year. He managed to stop payment on his check but he forgot about the two credit cards until the next billing period when he noticed charges against both cards by nonhospital personnel. This of course entailed dozens of phone calls before finally the charges were removed. The story, gruesome as it was, was not unique. Everyone had a favorite, ready for the telling.

Of course there are also stories from the other end of the spectrum: mangled lumps of humanity, mutilated into anonymity, deposited by ambulance into the tender mercies of faceless medical technicians. Weeks, months, sometimes years later the incredible results are detailed in newspaper or magazine human-interest stories. A life restored, a spirit reconstructed. A tearful testimonial: "No words could ever express my gratitude to the doctors and nurses." But for every such heart-warmer, there are tens of horror stories. On the streets of a big city, the odds, it's fair (or maybe unfair) to say, very definitely do not favor the casual victim of crime, accident, or mishap.

Yet the odds broke marvelously in Jack's favor. Police within seconds blocked the street, diverting northbound traffic away from Jack's fallen form. A city ambulance appeared and within half an hour Jack was carried into the emergency room of St. Vincent's Hospital at West Twelfth Street and Seventh Avenue.

Patrick Boland, surgeon-extraordinaire, a loyal son of Eire who returned to the Old Country every year to do pro bono work in a Dublin hospital, was just completing a sixteen-hour shift. He was on his way home. But there was a patient just brought into the emergency room. Would he take a look?

Both Jack and I have had more than our fair share of good luck. But no chunk of rosy luck surpassed that early morning moment when Patrick Boland sighed, shrugged, and said, "Why not?"

In X-ray Jack's femur was shown to have splintered in four places. Extensive internal bleeding surrounded the injury. He'd suffered a brain concussion. Shock had set in. Vital signs were worrisome. Overall condition was deemed critical. The accepted medical protocol called for surgery to align the fragmented bone, multiple blood transfusions to compensate for blood loss, and finally the application of a plaster cast that would extend from the armpits down over the right leg, all the way to the ankle. It was a protocol that would require the patient to remain horizontal for a minimum of four to six weeks. At the end of that time, provided that healing was sufficiently advanced, therapy would begin. If all went well, the patient could hope to achieve full, or as full as possible, recovery within a year. It was fairly straightforward and certainly the generally accepted method of procedure. Nothing, needless to say, is foolproof, and in cases such as Jack's, there remained one very major hazard: pneumonia. Being forced to remain horizontal for weeks on end invited, some would even say ensured, the accumulation of fluid in the lungs, with pneumonia following as a natural consequence.

Patrick Boland chose an alternate route. Four hours on the operating table. Minuscule shards of bone were removed. The other fragments were secured to a metal shaft by screws. The incision was closed. No cast was prescribed. The objective was to restore the integrity of the leg without depriving the body as a whole of vital functions both circulatory and muscular. As for the concussion, just give it time. By mid-afternoon Jack was sleeping off the anesthetic in a room high above Seventh Avenue. Mark, Jenny's brother, summoned from his Manhattan copyediting desk, hovered nearby. To Jenny had fallen the task of tracking me down. And so she had.

His leg, I thought. Thank God, just his leg. Legs had no brains, no powers of discernment, no sense of humor or analytical powers. Jack, I told myself, would still be Jack, a realization that made me weak with relief.

Across all the distance that lay between us I wrapped my arms around Jenny's shoulders. I held her close and breathed my tangled prayers of gratitude into that warm place where neck curves softly into bone. Tomorrow, we told each other. I'll be there tomorrow. As soon as I know, I'll call you. No, don't even think of meeting me. I'll take a cab and come straight to the hospital. Has she had a chance to tell the rest of the family? Does everyone know? Tell everyone that I'm . . . I'm what? On my way? Not exactly. Not yet. No. I was just sitting over here an ocean away, about as useless as a human being could possibly be.

If only I could have clung to Jenny all that night, never hanging up the phone, but of course she had her own concerns—the immediacy of being with her father, of rearranging our respective lives to accommodate Jack's accident. Medical insurance, patient ID, notifying the *Times*, even retrieving the bike that, against all odds, remained just where the cops had placed it, leaning against a light post.

The next day in a state best described as numb, I took a direct flight from Bordeaux to Newark, a route that, thanks to its wonderful convenience, has long since been eliminated.

Not Jenny but Cathy was there, having bamboozled her way past security checkpoints so as to stand right by the doorway through which we poured into the terminal.

"I said *not* to meet me," I told her, holding her fast in a bear hug. "Didn't Jenny tell you?"

"Of course she told me. But we agreed to pay no attention."

I didn't want to let go. "I'm so glad, so glad!"

No waiting for luggage. I'd hauled everything aboard with me to avoid any delay. Together we made it arm in arm out to the parking lot and there in the privacy of the car, I had to gather her in all over again, grateful for the ten millionth time for the blessing of family. Seeing her there, so composed and lovely, radiating not just health and youth but a quiet kind of reassurance, lifted my spirits. A huge overdose of fatigue seemed to melt away.

As we navigated out of the airport, through the Lincoln Tunnel and downtown to the hospital, Cathy brought me up to date. The surgery was successful. Jack was out of recovery and in his own room. Last night he was pronounced "stabilized." Pause.

We threaded our way through a patch of tricky traffic, trucks loading and unloading. A stalled car with a tiny, hapless Asian woman behind the wheel, her panic rising as impatient cabs let loose a blast of horns.

Finally clear, I waited for the next news bulletin. But none came.

"So is that what he is now?" I asked. "Stabilized?"

"Well, that's what he was last night. About six. But . . ."

"But what?"

"Well, some time around midnight, he had a slump."

"A slump? Like what?"

"They said it wasn't all that unusual. His blood pressure dropped. He seemed to have some trouble breathing. There was some talk of putting him into intensive care. But then he rallied. This afternoon, he seems much better. Good color. He's eating."

"Just like that he came around? All on his own?"

"Not completely on his own."

"What does that mean?"

Cathy maneuvered up beside a pickup truck and deftly passed it, zipping through a light just as it was turning. A good city driver. Once again in the clear, she glanced over at me for just an instant before replying.

"They thought he was having a reaction, I guess you'd call it a delayed reaction, to the blood he lost." Another pause. "So early this morning they gave him a transfusion."

"How much of a transfusion?" Half-formed fears of AIDS floated along the edges of my thoughts.

As if reading my mind, Cathy quickly added, "Don't worry about the blood. They assured us it was completed screened. You know, for hepatitis, for AIDS, for whatever else you have to watch out for."

I breathed out a long anxious breath. "Well, that's something, I suppose."

"Of course it's something. It's better than something. It's a godsend!"

"You're right. Certainly. How much blood did they give him?"

"Just two pints."

"Two pints. That's not so much, is it?"

"No, it's not. And look at it this way. Those two pints probably saved his life."

"And what about the concussion?"

"They say, just give it time."

"That's all?"

"Evidently."

I let out a deep sigh of relief. We exchanged a long look of hope and sunny optimism.

*

That was the spring and summer devoted to healing. Within a week Jack was home. Mobility meant at first a walker, and pretty soon crutches. No weight bearing on the broken leg before September. But every day, from Memorial Day weekend onward, we went to the salt water pool of our nearby beach club. There, with skillful maneuvering of his crutches, Jack was able to make it down the four steps into the water. With slow, steady strokes he would make it back and forth, down the length of the pool, staying within arm's reach of the edge. Just in case. But all went well. Whatever pain there was seemed manageable with nothing more than over-the-counter remedies. Our days fell into a pleasant routine—newspapers read from page one all the way through, books consumed, four or five a week.

It was a year with plenty to think about. Nelson Mandela walked out a free man after more than twenty-seven years in prison and the Supreme Court said it was okay to burn the flag. Bad man Saddam Hussein marched into Kuwait to claim its oil. The U.S. Marines swooped into Panama and in a very messy operation nabbed Manuel Noriega, which prompted President George Bush to tell us how big a victory had been won in the war against drugs. Stefan Edberg took Boris Becker to five sets before he was able to hoist some twenty pounds of engraved silver on the center court at Wimbledon, and Martina Navratilova did no less for the women, locking up that title for the third time. Here at home Pete Sampras overcame André Agassi, his serve as well as his histrionics, to win his first U.S. Open. The Cincinnati Reds won the World Series.

It was also Jack's fiftieth Harvard reunion. Never one to tarry over sentimental moments, he had, nonetheless, planned to attend. When it became apparent that even with high-grade crutching skills, it still would be totally impractical, he shrugged it off, though we both admired the commemorative toys brought back by classmates. A perfectly decent coffee mug, complete with university insignia and class date. A handy pocket flashlight. And a fistful of alma mater solicitations with heavy emphasis on the tax advantage that would be his as soon as he dropped his check in the mail.

By September the crutches gave way to a cane. By October he was back on his bike, and well before Trick or Treat he was once again at his desk at the *Times*. I don't recall that we ever discussed or even mentioned either the concussion or those two pints of blood.

12

Alzheimer's disease is a progressive, degenerative and irreversible brain disorder that causes intellectual impairment, disorientation and eventually death. There is no cure. It is estimated that 2–5% of people over 65 years of age and up to 20% of those over 85 years of age suffer from the disease.

The exact cause of the disease is unknown. Alzheimer's disease is linked to gradual formation of plaques in the brain, particularly in the hippocampus and adjoining cortex.

BBC World Service, http://news.bbc.co.uk

A few years ago I read an article by a woman who held an important, high-level government job. She was in good health, sound of mind and body as the phrase goes. Then after half a century of everything going along smoothly, her life began to unravel. Her husband of many years died. Her only daughter divorced and soon moved from the East to the West Coast. Maybe there were some other things that went awry that I've forgotten. I do remember, however, that she had to undergo serious and extensive dental work that for some reason or other did not turn out the way it should have. She began to sink into a depression. Her workday no longer slid by effortlessly. Mistakes began cropping up in her work. Within the year, everything seemed to be falling apart for her. She consulted with her regular doctor who referred her to a psychiatrist, and she found herself confronting a rather horrendous recommendation: she should consider, said the doctors, undergoing electroshock therapy for the depression. She did what any intelligent person would do under the same circumstances. She got a second, and maybe a third, opinion. She did some layman research on the effects of electroshock and in the end, reluctantly, she agreed to the prescribed treatments.

Her recovery was "uneventful." After a brief period of time she was cleared to return to her job. Her daily work required exactitude as well as some math. Work that she had handled effortlessly for years suddenly was beyond her mental capability. It wasn't just that she had forgotten essential data—she had been warned about possible short-term memory loss—but even when the data were provided she found herself unable to process it. Her superiors were considerate, and no deadline was set for her work to come up to scratch. But after trying for a reasonable period of time— several months, maybe a year—she had to admit that she was no longer capable of doing the work that she had handled for decades. Her conclusion remains vivid in my mind. Had her work not required a relatively high level of mental function, she said, she would have had no reason to question her full recovery. Daily life, social relationships, paying her bills, and maintaining contact with her daughter could all be managed just as before the treatment. It was only the exacting requirements of her job that enabled her to understand that her mental functions had been permanently, substantially, and irreversibly diminished.

At the time that I read that account I thought how most of us can manage our lives without ever imposing strenuous cerebral demands on ourselves. Daily life unfolds day by day by routines into which we can usually settle with relative ease. Were we to be deprived of, say, twenty or forty percent of our cognitive abilities, would we even be aware of that deprivation? Unless, like the woman whose poignant account I read, we were confronted with mentally demanding work, chances are we would act and sound just like our usual selves.

I have also read that our brains generate more than 200 billion neurons that depend on more than fifty chemical transmitters by which thought, sensation, instinct, emotion, and a wealth of other undefined reactions travel across trillions of dendrites and axons with a speed that, for the layman at least, is simply termed "faster than instantaneous."

Stricken in the fall, Jack had, by early summer, largely recovered his coordination. He tired very easily. Still he was able to converse with Mark, who stopped in several times a week, bringing news of his steadily expanding writing career in the field of sports books for juveniles. Maybe "converse" is not quite the exact word. But he made a strenuous effort to be attentive. He would ask a question or two, but gone was his real self that would have sought all kinds of details about the work in progress, would have wanted to know, "What's next?" There had never been a time in either Mark's or Jenny's life that Jack had failed to take immeasurable pride in their accomplishments. That pride was undiminished, but the mental agility to sustain it was gone. In its place was a kind of passivity that seemed so at odds with his true self. It was that passivity as much as anything else that made me realize, no matter how reluctantly, just how deep were the inroads made by the disease.

I had neither the means nor the inclination to measure whatever erosion was taking place. One day folded into another. All my efforts were directed toward keeping life simple, unruffled, as free of complications as possible. What Jack was able to do one day and unable or unwilling to do the next could be attributed to so many variables—weather, fatigue, the distraction of comings and goings in the household. I had no interest in ascribing cause and effect. What couldn't be managed today—scanning the morning paper, opening the day's mail, placing a phone call, with the number written clearly and in bold print beside the phone—could doubtless be managed tomorrow, or the next day. Only reluctantly and after weeks or even months, did I come to accept that a task postponed today, would soon drop off the Things He Can Do List. Permanent deletions.

The ways of the medical profession are not so loosely structured. Though the root causes of Alzheimer's may remain a mystery, though little is understood about how and why it progresses as it does, still in the world of the health maintenance organization there are niceties to be observed. The physician–patient relationship can be defined as comforting on one end, lucrative on the other. And what did we know? Wasn't there always the off-chance that something would emerge that could actually stem the progress of the disease? Even reverse damage already done? So we elected to "stay in touch."

The decor in Dr. X's offices was Williamsburg Sterile. Pale greens and blues.

Beige underfoot. The lighting adequate but not alarming. The chairs orthopedically correct and acceptably comfortable. Plenty of *National Geographic*s, not too tattered. We went on a ninety-day basis just to see "how we are getting along." Driving from home to the office I would touch on the subjects that I knew would loom front and center. "It's May such and such or June such and such," I'd say.

"Of course," Jack would say. "I know that."

"I know you do. And I bet you know our address as well."

Sometimes he did. If not all of it, at least parts of it. Maybe the name of our lane, or the name of our town. As for the zip code, he'd never much bothered with zip codes anyway so why start now? Questions of national events, the name of the president, for instance. Never in doubt. The year? Here a muddle. Time had lost its proper sequence. It could be the 1960s, the 1980s, sometimes the 1940s. His age too had lost its context. He only rarely hit on the right number of years.

We would sit together in the waiting room. To allay a possible burst of impatience from Jack I would try to keep his attention engaged with nonstop inconsequentials. The weather. The national scandal or the international disaster of the day. I found myself squirreling away jokes, grandchildren anecdotes, news of friends, saving them for just such in-between waiting periods. On one occasion I rose from my chair, crossed the room to select a magazine and, on turning back, I found Jack pulling on his coat, heading for the door. Catching up with him I laid a hand on his arm, a gesture to delay or forestall departure. In perfectly amicable fashion he looked down at me and said, "What? Can't we go?"

"Not until we've seen the doctor," I said quietly.

It gave him pause. A puzzled expression claimed his features.

"The doctor? Haven't we seen him? Isn't that over?"

"Not yet. In just a few minutes. Then we'll be on our way."

Without protest he returned to his seat.

"I thought we were all finished," was his only comment.

*

"Shall we start with the clock?"

It was, of course, rhetorical. We always started with the clock.

Unable to offer remedy or cure, the medical community has devised procedures by which at least a patient's decline can be measured. Theirs is a better-than-nothing approach. Send no one away empty-handed.

The routine never varied. Dr. X would hand Jack a yellow legal pad, a pen, and a request that he draw a clock, the hands indicating twenty minutes before four. Was that exact time stipulated by multimillion dollar research programs? Did white-coated savants in gleaming labs hit upon that time only after testing hundreds, maybe thousands of unsuspecting humans for whom the face of a clock was rapidly losing all relevance?

A lefty, taught to write with his right hand, Jack's artistic capabilities had always been about as close to zero as a sophisticated level of literacy would permit. Thirty years ago, his artistic rendition of a clock would doubtless have been a hasty scrawl. He was a man of words, not designs. So a lopsided circle would appear on the lined yellow sheet. Pause. A half gesture to lay the pad back on the desk would be interrupted with an encouraging word or two to include the numbers and the hands of the clock. Hesitantly, Jack would fill in the numbers, not always legibly. And what import if they spilled over the rim of the clock? Again, an effort to hand back the pad. "Now place the hands at twenty minutes of four."

The windows in that office were set high in the wall. Treetops in a smother of greens or naked and gleaming, encrusted in ice, were all that could be seen. Early on I learned to turn windowward, oh so engrossed in all that arboreal profusion.

The doctor's tone was level, firm, not unkind. Professional. A careful exchange of phrases: on your way out, see my secretary, an appointment, shall we say eight weeks?

I matched him, stiff smile for stiff smile. My nods, thanks, murmured assents followed us like a vapor trail down the hall to the receptionist's desk.

13

In normal aging, we also experience everyday lapses in communication and memory, as well as regular destruction of "tired" brain cells. These everyday lapses, nonetheless, do seem worrisome, because who can tell whether they are the early signs of Alzheimer's or just "normal aging"? Some scientists have theorized that the common, everyday lapses of normal aging are the happy result of a "pruning" process, wherein our mature brains discard the insignificant details of an idea or event, and retain only the import "gist" or "essence" of that idea or event.

www.lifestages.com/health/alzheime.html

Molly O'Brien, R.N., was promoted up and out of white starchy uniforms and ugly white shoes to senior visiting nurse. She would arrive in pretty scarves, elegant pants, her glorious abundance of chestnut hair subdued by a gold hair band or a bit of black velvet ribbon. She was a delight. All of her professionalism was firmly tucked away, out of sight, hidden under a veneer of cheery hellos and smiles that would have dispelled clouds across all of her native Killarney. I could count on the fingers of one hand the good things that had befallen us since Jack fell ill. Of these, Molly O'Brien was worth two, maybe three of those fingers.

Our medical circumstances required a nurse or equivalent to stop by once a month, just to make sure all was on the up and up.

Really? I asked Molly. Did anyone ever fake debilitation? Were there supposedly homebound people who sneaked out to shoot a round of pool, wager a wad on the daily double, or cadge a joint in the town park? Had Molly actually come across Alec Guinness–type scoundrels happily collecting illegal benefits while posing as invalids? Out of dressing gowns and into tweed and flannel, off to enjoy life somewhere out there beyond the clutches of insurance companies and HMOs.

"Well, you'd be surprised," was Molly's laughing reply. "Which is exactly why I'm here to see that everyone is on the straight and narrow."

Even Jeff was happy to greet her, cavorting around her, exuding delight when she bent to scratch behind his ears. "Mr. Jefferson," she'd say, "Are you looking after everything?" Jeff would bound ahead of her leading the way to where Jack waited in the living room.

A deft check of vital signs. Good appetite? Getting out for a bit of fresh air, are we? Keeping an eye, I hope, on this wife of yours. No telling what she might be up to. And unfailingly she would have Jack laughing. Always a pushover for a pretty face, a winning way, he would seem to return from the far-off landscape in which he wandered with increasing frequency.

As often as I could, I would slip away to leave Molly alone with Jack. I did so not just in the name of privacy, though that was certainly part of it. But without my hovering presence Jack had no other option but to answer Molly's questions unaided, something he avoided when he could.

It was after one of Molly's visits, a day in autumn when yellow leaves were twirling down like paper airplanes and the air was tinged with bronze, we were strolling, she and I, to where she'd parked her car in the driveway.

"What a pleasure of a man," she said, "even now when so much is slipping away."

"Well put," I told her. "A pleasure of a man."

"I asked him how the two of you came to meet."

"Oh-h?"

I opened the car door and held it wide for her.

She swung in with an easy grace that survived two decades of marriage and five children, the oldest not yet out of high school.

"He told me how you two first met. He said in Hanoi. Can that be so? What took him there? Or, more to the point, what took you there?"

I stopped abruptly, the car door poised to slam shut. Something must have shown on my face, some expression of bewilderment from my cocked and inquisitive eyebrow.

"Or perhaps I misunderstand," she added, not pressing the point.

I faltered, then groped for words of refutation, dismissive words by which to lightly gloss over what surely had to have been some delusional lapse on Jack's part.

"I can't imagine," I began and then in one of those sleight of hand tricks that time can play, memory whirled backwards and I regained my footing.

"Yes," I told her. "He's right. Well, at least, in a manner of speaking he's right. I guess you could say, we did meet in Hanoi. In a way."

I offered no further explanation. Nor was any asked.

For the briefest instant she laid a hand firmly on mine. A nod, a quick smile, and she was gone.

*

On the third floor of the Lincoln Building, overlooking Madison Avenue, I'm at my desk, a wooden splintery affair, drawers down the left side, a not-too-secure leg on the right side. The surface is buried under heaps of folders. Not sensible ring binder folders or fold-over folders with a dab of Velcro to guarantee sanity. Of course not. These are French folders. Meager manila things crammed with handfuls of tissuey pages. I've learned to hold body and soul together with elastic bands. Of the four in this office, I am the only American. No one else depends on elastic bands. Or paper clips for that matter. Rather everyone but me depends on a time-honored technique: tap-tap pages into alignment. Fold down the top left corner. Then deftly tear two small cuts half an inch apart and with a quick twist of the wrist, press the cut backward and voilá—fail-safe order. I've tried it, without success.

At least once a day a stack of folders begins to slide. Invariably I'm tethered to the phone, helpless to interrupt the cascade. Everyone understands. Smiles, shrugs, maybe a helpful hand to retrieve the slippery pages. And once again we're all reminded that my American modus operandi is hopelessly inadequate in this little hive of French busyness.

Michèle, Simone, Monsieur Hayatt, and me. Michèle is the office typist. She spends much of the day on the phone. Her life is difficult. She lives with François, an Algerian guitarist who plays all night at a club down on East Fourteenth Street. He sleeps through the day. Michèle must call at frequent intervals to rouse him for chores that can't await her return. She calls to remind him to "*décrochez le Meester Café.*" Or "*N'oubliez pas Bibi. Il manque de l'eau frais.*" Their life is complicated. Bibi is an illegal parrot, one of a succession, smuggled in by a friend from North Africa in tennis ball cans. The friend offloads them to pet shops in Brooklyn and Queens for astonishing prices. Michèle and François help out as sort of foster parents for parrots not yet sold. It's a setup that I think parallels "parking stock," a Wall Street practice that is evidently illegal but not uncommon. Michèle has tightly permed blond curls and an expression of bone-deep lassitude. It's not clear to me whether her duties as typist include typing correspondence for me. I'm hesitant to ask. So rather than take a chance, I type my own letters, using up a bottle of Wite-Out a week.

Simone is small with short dark hair, as pretty, as sleek as a red-winged blackbird. Even in darkest December her skin keeps a warm Mediterranean glow that suggests lemons, olives, and sun-splashed terra cotta walls. Not even the sickly light of the overhead fluorescent lights (Aren't such lights supposed to be unhealthy, causing eye damage, or is it cancer? Haven't the French heard? Why are they not more up on such matters?) can diminish the luminosity of Simone's lovely face. All of Simone's gestures are deft, sure. The flip of a lid from a coffee cup, the handwritten memos in a script perfected in childhood's French cahiers under the eye of state-appointed professors. From the knees up Simone is all grace and competence. But her left leg ends in a heavy black shoe that balances on a six-inch platform. To lift it she has to swing her hip high. It hurts even to watch. As if to compensate for the treacherous left foot, she invariably wears a fragile something on the right foot—a slingback bit of patent leather, a brazenly high heel, open-toed in summer, insubstantial in all seasons. How does she manage the daily crush, hurrying up and down the steps of the subway, which she rides daily to and from work? Had she been born in New York instead of Lyons, would that left foot have been repaired in infancy when the bones were soft and pliable? It is just one more France–U.S. quandary by which I'm forever beset.

Among us, Michèle, Simone, and I, Monsieur Hayatt is indisputably Alpha. He is a French-speaking Egyptian Jew, a hopeless ethnic brew. He has the round, brown, pock-marked face of a gingerbread man just baked and lifted out to cool. And like a gingerbread man, there is a hapless quality about him. The slope of his portly shoulders, the doleful cast of his hooded eyes, his gesture of casting both hands wide, palms up, an acting-school ploy denoting despair—all portray a scapegoat, someone born to suffer for the idiocy of others. Even on those rare occasions when he laughs, a dry, hollow sound, it is evident that he has no faith in the moment's humor.

All day long Monsieur Hayatt sits tipped back in his ancient swivel chair, his head of thinning, pomaded black hair dipping dangerously close to the floor. The telephone is his only confidante. Into it he murmurs hour after hour. Occasionally I catch a French word or two but whether for the most part he is speaking English, Arabic, French or maybe even some other language to which he never admits, I have no way of knowing. Furthermore, I am at pains in actuality and in appearance not to intrude. Before I was brought into the office and installed at my splintery desk in the corner, Monsieur Hayatt had this smallish space all to himself. His privacy was absolute. His supremacy unchallenged. It was an office for one. But now we are two and his hot humiliation is clearly palpable. I am here by order of "*la diréction*" in Paris. In the face of such august authority we both are helpless.

We quickly adapt. Like the Japanese, constrained from birth by lack of space, taught to bow, hands at the side, always remaining rigidly within an undeclared but clearly perceived allocation of space, Mr. Hayatt and I come and go in scrupulous orbits, carefully designed never to intersect.

"Bonjour, Monsieur," I murmur on entering the office in the morning. He is always there ahead of me. I avert my eyes in a vain effort to afford him maximum privacy. I speak in a modulated voice so as not to intrude on his telephone dialogue.

A hasty glance in my direction and then, "Bonjour, Madame." Instinctively he hunches forward, swivels around, cups a gingerbread hand around the mouthpiece of the phone and resumes his murmured monologue.

It's the behavior of someone who is pouring out his heart to a patient, doubtless loving listener. But what do I know? Perhaps this is business conducted *à la française*. As best I understand it, Monsieur Hayatt is concerned with French textbooks, their sales, their shipping, their storage in warehouses the whereabouts of which seems always to be in doubt.

Do American schools use many textbooks published in France? I would doubt it. Isn't it a given that American schoolchildren must receive their second language in very gentle sips? What American fourth grader could withstand the steely-eyed rigors of a French schoolmaster holding aloft an honest to God French textbook?

Perhaps, I wonder—though not often and not for long—these textbooks are being ordered and read by French schools, a handful of lycées where the sons and daughters of foreign diplomats, Middle Eastern sheiks, and deposed royalty pursue their lessons in a rarefied atmosphere uncontaminated by Drivers' Ed, Band Practice, and Family Hygiene.

My morning routine varies hardly at all. I hang my coat on the back hook of the tippy wooden square shaft of a coat rack (circa 1910) leaving the other three hooks for Monsieur Hayatt. I do not presume.

I take my seat and thank Simone for handing over my list of phone calls and my *"courrier."* I have no problem with the letters from U.S. publishers. The letters from Paris are more demanding. There are phrases, coined no doubt by Napoleon, that must be sprinkled liberally through even the simplest of transactions. Of course, the closing phrases date all the way back to Louis XIV and far be it from me to abbreviate.

"Please accept, kind sir, the assurance of my most respectful homage."

"Will you rest assured of my most sincere gratitude for your attention, dear sir, to this matter at hand."

In a drawer I keep a list of these phrases, trying to remember the subtle hierarchal gradations by which one is to be preferred over another. My lot would be considerably eased if I could simply refer the occasional quandary to Monsiur Hayatt: *"Veuillez m'expliquer, Monsieur?"* But the entrenched customs by which we both abide forbid such intimacy.

It's a kind of truce, a wall of glass that, barring unforeseen circumstances, can endure indefinitely. But unforeseen circumstances burst in upon us, out of the nowhere into the here: The 1967 Israeli–Egyptian Six-Day War.

I arrive on a Monday morning. At once I see that all rules are suspended. Michèle is not on the phone. Nor is she typing. Rather, she and Simone are conversing earnestly, with unmistakable urgency. With frequent furtive glances they keep tabs through the open doorway on Monsieur Hayatt. Trouble, as tactile as summer lightning, crackles through the room. Apprehensive, I walk on through the outer office to the shared space beyond.

"Bonjour," I begin. But I get no further. Monsieur Hayatt sits deep in his chair, tipping forward, his elbows on his knees and his huge head held tenderly between his palms.

"Chère Madame."

He extends one hand. Incredulity and astonishment all but overcome me. Anxious not to fall short of what he expects, or needs, or hopes for, I step up awkwardly and take his hand in both of mine. He continues, his voice faltering, and it becomes apparent, even to my obtuse American sensibilities, that we have emerged, Monsieur Hayatt and I, onto the broad but unfamiliar landscape of friendship. To my astonishment, I'm being addressed not just as a friend but as a friend whose arrival confers a generous measure of relief. In long, shuddering sighs he pours out his woes, each word a thread in the bond of confidentiality he weaves between us. His family, he tells me, is stranded in Cairo. Behind locked doors. The shutters closed and fastened. No telephone. No electricity. At any moment the artillery shells will fall. Perhaps poison gas. "*Madame, vous n'imaginez pas leur terreur!*" As I listen it occurs to me that if it takes a war to dissolve the froideur between us, then as far as I'm concerned, the war is well worth it.

The war was brief. As was his distress. The Israelis achieved a breakthrough, not just in the sands of the Sinai but also in our little outpost devoted to the promotion of *les livres scolaires*. Decorum returned. But from that day forward Mr. Hayatt and I existed on a plateau of amiable even cordial relations.

*

"Just what is it that you do?"

It's a question I'm asked not infrequently and I know perfectly well that before the question mark is even in place, the attention of the inquisitor is already drifting off to something more arresting on the conversational horizon.

"I'm the U.S. representative for a French publisher. For sale and purchase of book rights between France and the U.S."

"Oh-h-h?" with an almost imperceptible quickening of interest. "And just exactly what . . ."

"I sell the rights to books published in France to U.S. publishers and, conversely (I never omit conversely) I buy for the French market the rights to books published over here."

"Really?" And at once I'm elevated to a new and altogether pleasing level of respect. In truth the job description I provide is correct. It would hold up in any court of law. But the gap between the description and actuality is Grand Canyon huge. The reason for the disparity rests squarely in the cultural gulch that separates France from the U.S.

To begin with, U.S. publishers have minimal interest in books published in France. To judge by their attitudes, one would assume that French literature ground to a halt with Sartre, de Beauvoir, and Camus. Of course, the greats continue in print— Voltaire, Hugo, Flaubert, Balzac, Baudelaire, Proust—reissued year after year in bindings befitting the classics. But after Proust . . . *le Grand Silence.*

To be fair, it's not a case of yawning disinterest on the part of U.S. publishers. Rather, it is a case of too few U.S. editors bothering to read French books with the intention of giving them a thoughtful evaluation. And if this is true of French writing, and it is, then imagine how little hope there is for German, Arabic, Portugese,

Italian, Chinese, Japanese, or any other foreign literary efforts. Our insularity is by no means confined exclusively to our geography. Let's face it, we are a hopelessly monolingual tribe.

On that rare occasion when a French book surfaces that is adjudged a good bet in the U.S. market, it still must overcome a formidable hurdle. Unless a British publisher is willing to share fifty-fifty the cost of translation, the contract will remain unsigned.

The French, on the other hand, evince an insatiable appetite for U.S. writers. Not just Hemingway, James Jones, and James Baldwin, all ex-pat Parisians, but also Updike, Willa Cather, Bellow, Faulkner, Mary McCarthy, Vonnegut, Eudora Welty—all are familiar names in millions of French households. You would think that would mean lots of busy work for someone like me. Not so. All these authors are already represented by diligent literary agents who would never dream of letting the foreign rights of their writers' books be traded by the publisher. Not when the agent's alternative is to negotiate those rights at the annual book fair in Frankfurt, Germany. Why should they discuss that sale with me, closeted over there in my Madison Avenue cubbyhole, when they could instead discuss it over brandy and soda in the cozy brass and leather bar of the Frankfurterhof?

So with one half of my responsibilities rendered more or less moot, I'm left with the other half, which is entertaining but nonproductive. An exciting series of new math textbooks, K-12, has just been brought out, endorsed by an impressive committee of educators in California. Would the French be interested in taking a look? A line of YA (young adult) books is being launched in the fall. In France there are no Young Adults. French youth moves from moppethood directly into the ranks of scholar with few stops in between.

Sample copies of U.S. books pile up around my desk, delivered by publishers who dwell forever in the land of useless optimism. Dutifully I look them over, complete the evaluation form provided by the head office in Paris, and send them on across the sea in the office pouch dispatched Par Avion every Friday afternoon.

It's rare that these titles or their authors are ever mentioned again. Instead, Paris responds with an elaborate sales program by which I am asked to sell the rights to a six-volume series for children on the life of Napoleon. Volumes I and II are already in print: Napoleon's childhood. Volumes III to VI will be off the press shortly. Can Madame please propose the series to major U.S. textbook publishers and let Paris know "*hors et delá*," that is, ASAP, when the enclosed sales contract will be signed. It's not difficult to appreciate the degree to which my job, while sounding challenging and rewarding, was, in fact, a triumph of futility.

It's a Friday in the spring. On Madison Avenue the rain is coming down in torrents. The wind is tipping trash cans and street signs are swinging back and forth in alarming arcs. If I leave by quarter of four, I can catch the shuttle across town, the Seventh Avenue subway down to Penn Station, and the 4:30 train home. To that end I attempt to corral the day's correspondence, tuck books-to-be-read-this-weekend into my take-home satchel. When the phone rings, I hesitate. If I don't pick up, Simone will take the call and whatever it is I can put it off until after the weekend. I lean out to see what's what in the adjacent office. Simone is not to be seen and Michèle is huddled over the current *Marie-Claire*.

The phone continues to ring and with no help in sight, I answer it. The voice is urgent. Explanatory introductions are minimal. A man from the *New York Times* book publishing program. A new book by Harrison Salisbury. Time is of the essence. The subject? Hanoi. The French, the voice tells me, will surely be interested.

The hands of my desk clock are edging past the half hour.

Why don't you send it over, I say without much enthusiasm. But that proposal is rejected out of hand.

"Look, why don't I just get it over to you right now. I can be there in ten minutes. No. Less."

It's such an absurd suggestion. On a Friday afternoon? Late. In the pouring rain?

"Monday would be fine . . ." I begin but I'm too docile by half. Before I can muster my protests, I'm told "Just hold on. I'll be right there."

In our office visitors were neither expected nor welcome. Our contacts with "out there" were strictly by phone and by mail. If actual contact was deemed essential, either Monsieur Hayatt or I would venture forth to meet intruders before the first lines of defense were breached. Our little world, population of four, was far too insular to welcome intruders, even when they appeared, gifts in hand.

He arrives in a rush of words and raindrops, exuberance, impatience, and conviction emanating from him like static electricity. From a sodden manila envelope he draws forth the book, a slim volume, *Behind the Lines Hanoi*, by Harrison Salisbury. I know the background of the book. It has been favorably reviewed almost everywhere. The author, who had won a Pulitzer Prize for his reporting on the Soviet Union, had spent two weeks touring North Vietnam, its countryside, villages, and towns. What he saw was a far remove from what we at home were being told by our government. So-called pinpoint bombing was anything but. Viet Cong supply routes from north to south continued to function despite repeated raids by U.S. forces. Civilian casualties, according to the author, were a deliberate part of America's overall plan to break the enemy's spirit, to shatter the morale of the North Vietnamese. Although here at home we were being told emphatically and repeatedly that Hanoi was off-bounds for American bombing runs, Salisbury returned to write that bombs fell night after night on the city.

I haven't read the book, only the reviews. But already I am in sympathy with what Salisbury has to say. My feelings about what's happening in Vietnam are anything but complex. They are easily expressed, easily summarized: We shouldn't be there. We should get out. The sooner the better. But in the heat of discussion I can easily be overwhelmed with emotion, which only serves to defeat the cool, calm logic that would best serve my views. I examine the picture on the jacket of the tall, thin, bespectacled Yankee correspondent whose book this is, and think I'd be pleased to let this author speak for me as well.

Looming over me, the man who brought the book is speaking with enormous energy. His sense of urgency precludes any inclination on my part to interrupt. Raindrops drip onto my desk from the cuff of his extended sleeve. I glance sideways and notice that his raincoat is misbuttoned, a comic effect clearly at odds with the mission that brings him here.

"I'm sure the French will be interested in what Harrison has to say," he tells me. "After all, they have so many associations with Vietnam. Or do they still say Indochina?" I start to answer, but he closes me out. With an insistent finger, he taps the badly designed red, black, and gold cover of the book. "Pulitzer Prize-winning author, superb reporter, seven or eight previous books and all of them best sellers. This book is going to change a lot of thinking in this country." He pauses, steps back to see what effect his words have on me.

It is such a departure from the prototypical dialogue that should accompany transactions like this. Almost always when a publisher is proposing a title, he offers it along with a handful of other properties. It's the fall list or the spring list, and the merits of each title are neatly summarized; just right for persuading librarians and bookstore managers.

As I reach for a pen to take down the details—price, exclusivity of rights, Canada tossed in or reserved for the U.K.?—I glimpse Monsieur Hayatt, his face wreathed in astonishment and dismay. This sales pitch, unfolding in our circumspect little office, has no precedent. In the nanosecond that our eyes meet, he spins away, abashed to be caught eavesdropping. But I know his take on this odd encounter. In this too-small room there is too much energy, too much haste, and total disregard for the way matters such as this should be handled.

"So what do you think?"

Of course, it doesn't matter one whit what I think. The decision to buy or not buy is not mine to make. In fact, sometimes I think that a Yes recommendation from me in New York only invites a thumbs down from Paris. Furthermore, I know that there is not the slightest chance that the French will ever buy the book. Though Dien Bien Phu had fallen more than ten years ago, it was a name seared into the memory of every Frenchman. Now the Americans were going in to achieve where the French had failed? *Jamais de la vie!* What did the Americans know of the country? Did they know its history? Did they revere its literature, quote its poetry, admire its delicate artwork, savor its cuisine? Did they speak its singsong language, its words fragile as lace? Or understand its agrarian economy? Had they ever strolled the dykes between the rice-growing marshes, watched workers move from tree to tree tapping the lucrative juices to be processed into rubber? How many Americans had intermarried with the slim, elfin-like women who served their men with a devotion unimaginable in the land of fast food and drive-through everything?

Even the most disinterested Frenchman scoffed at the idea of American intervention. To the French, American defeat in Vietnam was a foregone conclusion, the sooner the better, and when it came no French tears would be shed.

Even the most disinterested Frenchman scoffed at the idea of American intervention. To the French, American defeat in Vietnam was a foregone conclusion, the sooner the better, and when it came no French tears would be shed.

But that is not the answer awaited by this tall, decidedly damp, clearly impatient man who stands between me and a reasonable Friday afternoon departure. "If you'll leave it with me, I'll get it read and have a report ready by Monday. Then I'll send it off to Paris the first of next week." He seems not to hear.

"I'll call you first thing Monday morning."

"Fine. But I won't have an answer by then."

"We could have lunch and talk it over."

"I'm not sure . . ."

"I'll call you. Monday. What time do you get in? Eight thirty? Nine?"

"Nine. Usually. But I could . . ."

"That's great. So I'll speak to you then."

He is already in the doorway, still dripping raindrops when he turns back and with no preamble, picks up a book tucked off on the far corner of my desk. My read-on-the-train book.

"She's marvelous, isn't she?" The "she" was Nadine Gordimer. The book was *Berger's Daughter*, the story of her early years in apartheid South Africa. "Til Monday, then."

As he makes once more for the door, he pauses just long enough to seize Monsieur Hayatt by the hand. "So nice to have met you," he says, and is gone.

As I wait in a fed-up-Friday mood for the 5:22, it comes to me with a start that I don't even know his name. Had he told me? Had I simply forgotten? Possibly. But I doubt it. Bumping down the gritty steps to the platform, overladen, off-balance, smothered in the go-home rush, I make an effort to recall the conversation. With only small success. I drop into the first empty seat and fish Harrison Salisbury's book from my sack. Perhaps there was a business card, some kind of a memo. I turn it over and study the author's face—a home-grown mustache, deep-set eyes, and an expression of sorrowful intelligence. Too bad. The book would die aborning on some remote desk in the warren of offices overlooking the Boulevard St. Germain. I lean my forehead against the cold, soot-streaked glass. My thoughts drift back to that hurried encounter. Such barely contained energy. The voice so charged with certainty. The raindrops dripping from his sleeve, blistering the letters on my desk. But a name? Blank. Just the raincoat, misbuttoned and hanging crooked. But even without a name, the recollection makes me smile. The man and this go-nowhere message from Hanoi.

And that, Molly O'Brien, was how we met.

14

Memory loss. Asking repeated questions. Trouble using words.
When signs like these begin to affect everyday life, they may not be a part of normal aging. They may be signs of Alzheimer's disease, an incurable progressive illness that robs patients and their families of a lifetime of memories. Today, however, the outlook for many is becoming more hopeful. ARICEPT is a clinically proven, once-a-day prescription medicine available to treat symptoms in patients with mild to moderate Alzheimer's disease. Already, over 860,000 patients in the United States have begun ARICEPT therapy. ARICEPT is well tolerated, but some people do experience side effects like nausea, diarrhea, insomnia, vomiting, muscle cramps, fatigue, and loss of appetite.

Drug advertisement for Aricept

All his life Jack was an addict. He was hooked on reading. Just as a smoker, given an unprogrammed moment, reaches reflexively for the pack, lighter, and matches, so would Jack reach for something to read. Newspaper, magazine, a book. The seams of his coat pockets were invariably split from having a book or maybe a whole newspaper shoved in, just in case. Just in case he had to wait five minutes for the gates to open, the plane to land, the curtain to go up, the game to start. History, biography, novels, political science, Le Carre, P. D. James, Freeman Dyson, John Mortimer, Tocqueville, Daniel Boorstin. He read three newspapers a day and who knows how many specialty newsletters.

Books piled up like autumn leaves beside the sofa, on window sills, atop his desk, atop his bureau, on the seats of the car, and of course in the bathroom, especially beside the tub where he loved nothing better than to soak for an hour, book in hand.

But now reading is out.

A huge black chasm of time has suddenly opened in his day. Still, habit prevailing, he would pick up a book. Within moments it would slip from his fingers. His eyes would lift from the page and even if I came along to read passages aloud to him, his gaze would wander and he'd stir restlessly, unable to focus.

It was during a phone conversation with the neurologist that I mentioned the woes that came with his inability to read. Surely it was nothing of which he was unaware. Wasn't this a common complaint, a typical syndrome of the disease? One would think. But only when I brought the matter up did he suggest we give Aricept a try. Five milligrams to begin with and if it was well tolerated, we'd up it to ten.

It's June. Jack was stricken the previous October. Not for eight months has he held a book or a newspaper to read all or even in part. Just how long was it after he started taking the two small yellow tablets that things changed? A week? Maybe two? Things moved slowly at first. It began with the morning newspaper. As always it was laid beside his plate at breakfast. Always left untouched. Then one perfect early summer day I watch him pick it up, scan the front page, and with a deft motion, fold the paper into fourths, subway style, turning to the editorial page. Such a simple, such an ordinary gesture. In an idiotic rush of feeling, it brings him back to me with a poignancy more properly reserved for acts of intimacy. Anxious that he not be disturbed, I take the phone off the hook. I intercept the mailman halfway to our door with a package too big for the roadside box. Silently I shoo Jeff outside lest he intrude with a wet black nose, seeking a bit of toast.

Over the next two weeks, just a few pages at a time, Jack makes his hesitant way into *A Perfect Storm* by Sebastian Junger. Not too bulky, not too long, decent print size, constructed in good, strong declarative sentences, evoking a bit of the New England coast that Jack knew well. It's fast-paced. Good research. An easy read.

It's a shirt-sleeve morning. We set out for our usual walk. To the bridge and back. By noon it will be hot. But Jack has put on not one but two sweaters, topped by the jacket of his good gray, pinstriped suit. His go-to-town suit. The day has long since passed when I try to referee his wardrobe. If I am with him when he dresses, the results are reasonably passable. If he dresses himself, no matter how inappropriately, my reaction is, So what. This is a so-what morning.

As we make our way, one slow step at a time, I talk about the book, referring to places and incidents, hoping to reinforce his tenuous hold on the story.

The Crow's Nest, the dockside bar and grill in Gloucester, Massachusetts, the same one that was so vividly described in the book. Only two years ago we, too, had hung out there one autumn afternoon, waiting for the skies to clear before boarding the sailboat of a friend. I tried to summon that afternoon to memory.

"Remember meeting Peter there that rainy afternoon? How we had lunch there? How the rains never let up? How we all talked so much we ended up staying on for supper? Remember the fisherman on the beach? The one who gave you that huge fish? How you took it, even though we were staying at the marina and had no place to cook it?

"Remember?"

Remember?

And of course, remembering is exactly what he can't do. If memory is the storehouse of all we've done, all we've been, then doesn't it follow that when memory vanishes, who we are must vanish, too?

We pause at the small bridge, our turnaround point. A flotilla of wild swans out in the river hangs motionless in a reedy cove, white plumage, green grass, blue-black water. A momentary miniature, just right for framing. In the clear, warm air, rich with the elemental smells of marshy mud and river water, we could hear the faint gabbling of the swans.

"Nice," I say, meaning the smells, the sounds, the moment.

"Yes. You're right. Really nice."

And for the next several steps, he walks if not lightly, at least more erect, less stooped, not quite so dependent on his arm around my shoulders or mine around his waist.

We are a little more than halfway home when out of the blue he says, "I wonder if he ever ran into Dmitri."

"He? Who?"

"The author. What's his name? Samuel? Simon?"

"Sebastian? Sebastian Junger?"

"Right. If he ever ran into Dmitri. While he was up there writing that book."

Dmitri? I am totally lost.

"He wore a yellow apron. He was Greek I think. Maybe Sicilian."

A yellow apron? Dmitri. Nothing, absolutely nothing comes to mind.

"I think you took a picture. Didn't you show me a picture of him, holding up a lobster, wasn't it you? Maybe it was someone else."

Yes! Yes! The lobsterman in Gloucester! He'd taken us both out one morning on his rounds to check his lobster pots.

I am elated. My heart thuds hugely against my ribs. One hand flies up to touch the quick warmth that flushes my cheeks. By what quirk has he come by this total recall?

But caution follows fast. Be still, be still I tell myself. As if even the beating of my heart could somehow undo whatever miracle is taking place.

We pause by our mailbox, next to an old swamp maple. We use it as a catch-your-breath tree, a place where Jack can rest his back, assess the distance back to the house and the safety of his chair by the window seat. The chair into which he'd drop, panting with exhaustion after even so brief an excursion.

As he stands propped by the tree, breathing hard, I lean back against him, ever so briefly. It's a stance repeated oh so often, always conveying to me something substantial, something absurdly protective and comforting. I take both his hands, the fingers cold despite the morning's warmth, and fold them in front of me. From my gut, reaching up shyly to the back of my throat, is a tendril of something immensely fragile, wondrously welcome. Hope.

Before nightfall I've described the morning's exchange to all our children. Over the phone I use words like "Breakthrough. His old self. Imagine his remembering that! And just think that was two, maybe three years ago." So many such phone calls had been wreathed in gloom, with nothing joyous to tell and nothing hinting of hope. Now to turn the tide, to call with something so positive, energizes and empowers me. At last, my turn to hand to all the family this chunk of something good.

He finished *The Perfect Storm*. It was the last book he ever read. All or in part. The paper, for the next week or so, scanned for a moment or two, then laid aside. One morning, hope spikes again when, bringing in a plate of buttered toast, I see him, so endearingly familiar, his reading glasses on his nose, the paper folded neatly, subway style held aloft, his eyes seemingly focused on the page. Only to see that he is holding it upside down. The big "breakthrough," the regeneration of powers lost, has come and gone in less than sixty days. So much for those once-a-day two small yellow pills.

15

People with one afflicted parent are 3 times more likely to develop Alzheimer's than those with no family history.

Newsweek, January 31, 2000, p. 50

Despite a fairly active agenda of clinical research, there is still no cure for Alzheimer's. Nor is there any conclusive evidence that families of most Alzheimer's victims are at any increased risk.

Alzheimer's: Late-Breaking Medical Research,
Center for Current Research, 1997 (Tel. 610-649-3165,
email: ccr@libertynet.org, Web site: www.lifestages.com)

Research on the cause of Alzheimer's is under way to determine whether it is inherited. It is not clear whether genetic factors are responsible.

www.nytimes.com/partners/microsites/from causetocure/
alzheimers/index.html

Jack was a history buff. In college he'd been encouraged and nourished by some formidable historians. Samuel Eliot Morrison and Daniel Boorstin were two he most enjoyed quoting. "The thing about history," he said to me more than once, "is that it's everywhere, all around you. It's right here under your nose."

"Uh-huh."

I suppose my responses were less than he'd hoped for, so on more than one occasion he felt compelled to prove his point. One such effort took him from the town dump, down a sandy twin-rut road that collapsed onto a small tidal island known as Barley Point. There, standing waist-high in the dune grass was a colony of shingled shacks, one-room affairs. No plumbing, no electricity. They were summer-only structures. The first islanders had been American Indians, probably Delawares.

They may have gathered reeds and rushes there, set snares for rabbits and prowled the island's shoreline for crabs and tasty mollusks but their nomadic ways precluded settling there. The first known householders built summer shacks there in the late 1800s and early 1900s. Most came from the outlying boroughs of New York City. Some were third- and fourth-generation summer residents. From our house it was only a ten-minute bike ride out to Barley Point. Once Jack discovered the island, he liked nothing better than to pedal out there early on a summer morning with Jeff delightedly trotting beside him, both on high alert for interesting tidbits. Over a cup of coffee or a frosty beer Jack heard how ownership had passed down through the generations, usually hand-me-downs from some long deceased relative—a grandparent, an old maiden aunt, a great-great uncle.

One especially gabby guy arrived every weekend from Queens with half a dozen kids in tow. "Leavin' the little woman at home to enjoy the peace and quiet." He told Jack he'd won his shack in a poker game. "A royal straight flush, hearts. Match that, I told them!" There were great yarns about September hurricanes and late May nor'easters; about the summer when grasshoppers stripped the island right down to the bone. "Not even a blade of grass left standing." There were hair-raising yarns about the good old bad days of Prohibition when bootleggers made fine use of the island's coves and its beaches sheltered by massive stands of cottonwoods and sea grape.

Invariably Jack would bike back home with tall tales to tell and often as not with a bluefish or a striped bass dangling from his handlebars, cheerfully oblivious to the fact that a just-caught fish is not the same as a fish scaled, gutted, and cleaned.

Whenever we would walk or bike to the beach, barely a mile, accompanied by inland grandchildren, Jack would insist that we pause to read aloud the inscription on a gray granite monument just before we crossed the drawbridge:

"On September 1, 1780, Captain Joshua Huddy was captured by a band of Tories. While being conveyed across the river to what is now Sea Bright, the boat was fired upon by Colonial forces. Although wounded, Captain Huddy escaped by jumping from the boat and swimming to the western shore. Subsequently he was captured by the British and hanged on April 12, 1782 at the Highlands."

The older children could manage with minimum help. The younger ones had no choice but to stand and listen, jiggling their buckets, squirming with impatience to get to the beach, the waves, and freedom. Crossing the bridge Jack would provide a thirty-second wrap-up of the American Revolution.

"And who do you suppose won?" he'd ask them. But already their sights were set on what lay ahead. It fell to me to say, "The British?"

*

Exploring the out-of-the-way. Jack was good at that. It was a talent that at one point in our lives we leaned on heavily.

On a hot, sticky New York evening, Jack drives by my office and picks me up, heading at scofflaw speed uptown. So where to this time? I ask. But already in the few weeks we've known each other, I've learned that the straightforward reply is not his style.

Why do you ask? Just know you'll love it.

In truth, I don't much care. The summer, the city, and us. That's enough.

City Island up in the Bronx is one of his favorites. The first time we go, he shows it to me as if he is the first explorer ever to set foot there.

"And I bet you never even knew it was here," he chortles. Somewhere along City Island Avenue, risking towing and fines, he locks the car, grabs my hand, and hustles me down through the summer dark to where Long Island Sound laps at our shoes. In front of us the black water wavers and bobs as if covered by colored cellophane—neon reds and greens, bug-repellent yellows, the reflection of onshore lights. Dinghys and sailboats, reduced in the night to ghostly hulls, fret audibly at their buoys, and cattails, against all the odds, poke up through the water in patches, land unwilling to give way to the sea. Way off along an invisible horizon the Triborough Bridge etches miniature scallops of incandescence against the night. The whole of the waterfront is edged with rickety docks, fish and bait shops, beer joints, and shingled shanties with doubtful front porches. The air is heavy with a mixture of smells—rotting vegetation and hot cooking oil bizarrely mixed with a layer of colder salty air that tastes as if it has blown in upon us from someplace far away. The whole place feels so unto itself, even though the sky behind us is luminous with the lights of Co-op City high rises.

On that first City Island expedition, seated outside at a splintery picnic table, contentedly making our way through a basket of fish and chips or fried clams or a bucket of shrimp, Jack remarks that we are dining in style in the land of the Siwanoy.

"The who?"

"The Siwanoy. Don't you know your pre-colonial history?"

"I guess not. I thought New York was all Algonquin or Mohawk."

"Not here on City Island. Here it was strictly the Siwanoy."

"How do you know?"

"I just know."

"I'm impressed." And I was.

"I knew you would be," with a wicked grin.

He laid claim not just to City Island but to a string of other places that belonged, however briefly, just to us. There was the cottage out on the Cape where rain leaked through the kitchen ceiling to splash neatly into the kitchen sink. In Ste. Maxime, just east of St. Tropez, there was La Belle Aurore, where our room hung out over the sea, even though we were told that at that time of year there was not a room to be had from Barcelona to the Italian border. There was the inn somewhere up the Hudson built of river stone, each stone worn so round and smooth that the whole place looked like mumps. Just one street down from the Seine there was the small hotel with a corkscrew for a staircase, and the breakfast tray, announced by a tap on the door, was discreetly placed on a table in the minuscule hallway.

The process by which we rearranged our lives was complex, lengthy, and expensive. Not that either of us thought it would be simple. I had three children. He had two. My children were just groping their way through adolescence into adulthood. Cathy was starting college, struggling heroically to keep her balance in the swirl of new experiences. Billy was in high school and Curt in junior high, absorbed in daily lives that precluded gazing much beyond the next quiz, the next game, the end of term.

Jack's children were considerably younger, Mark only seven and Jenny just three. How many times did we thrash the issue: Is it easier if they're older, or easier if they're younger? It was a debate that never came to a resolution.

I remember a friend, a confidante, having dinner with us once, well before we'd managed to glue the fragments of our lives together. She was a lawyer and a good one. She knew whereof she spoke. Referring to our respective situations she said, not with any great emphasis but simply to make a reasonable observation, "Whenever you have two failed marriages . . ." and Jack stopped her right there.

She looked up, surprised. "What?"

"I don't like that expression. Failed."

"Really?" She smiled but something in her expression said quite clearly she was not happy to be corrected.

"How would you put it, then?"

Jack paused thoughtfully and then said, very evenly, "I'd rather say unsuccessful. Not failed. Unsuccessful. That means it didn't work. That's all. It just didn't work."

I liked it better, too.

In one sense we were lucky well beyond our just deserts. Where children in a subsequent marriage can pose horrendous obstacles on the path of domestic tranquillity, ours brought not complications but delight. I had already survived the travails that go with children in elementary school, and so a second go-round held no terrors. Both Mark and Jenny were quick, bright, funny, and responsive. They were fun to be with. Nor did I ever lose sight of the fact that it was their father's loving pride in them and their devotion to him that eased his children's entry into our reconstructed lives. As for my own three children, they picked their own individual ways through a thicket of conflicting feelings that never alienated them from their father. And for that I was immensely grateful. Without ever thrusting himself into their lives, Jack won my children over by nothing more artful than simply being forever and ever himself. Uncritical, cheerful, never patronizing, and just as happy at the tennis court to take them on as partner or opponent. We were lucky. And we knew it.

16

Delusions are untrue ideas unshakably held by one person. . . . When delusions occur in a person who is known to have a brain impairment from strokes, Alzheimer's disease, or other conditions, the delusion is believed to arise out of the injury to brain tissue. It can be frustrating to have a person seem able to remember a false idea and unable to remember real information.

N. L. Mace and P. V. Rabins, *The 36-Hour Day*,
revised edition, Warner Books, 1992, p. 201

His two children were not the only bonus Jack brought to our newly united lives. He also brought a sizable coterie of friends that, gradually, over time, he passed along to me. They spanned multiple generations. They included do-away-with-the-government libertarians, communists-and-proud-of-it, actors, artists, pro football players, poets, pilots, playwrights, producers, down-and-outers, and many old college friends, some brilliant and some not so brilliant. Given their diversity, it seemed extraordinarily fortunate that with only one or two irrevocable exceptions, I enjoyed them all. Not too surprisingly, I had my favorites. In this category, no friends of Jack's earned my affection more speedily than the man he called "my godfather," a designation that bore no religious connotation. It was a term used between them to describe a rare brand of affection that each held for the other.

John Tunis was thirty years older than Jack. A hard-working journalist, author, avid sports fan, and lifelong tennis devotee, John found in Jack the son he never had. Their friendship began during Jack's freshman year at Harvard when the two met by chance at some Harvard varsity and junior varsity tennis matches. John was in the bleachers. Jack was on the court. Something about the left-handed, laid-back freshman with the corkscrew serve and an ability to shrug off bad calls that went against him attracted John, for whom sportsmanship was always and always a top priority. Gradually the friendship between the older man and the younger man ripened into a bond that held firm until John died at the age of eighty-five. By the time the two men met, the name John Tunis was already well known in the world of books, magazines, and international broadcasting. He was the first to make a trans-Atlantic broadcast of the tennis matches at Wimbledon for NBC. One of his best stories was how he made the broadcast from a perilous perch atop a tower of boxes, chairs, and stepladders, an improvised forerunner of today's luxurious press boxes.

His articles, usually but not always having to do with sports, both amateur and professional, appeared in the *New Yorker*, *Colliers*, the *Saturday Evening Post*, *Reader's Digest*, the *New York Times*, and in many metropolitan daily papers that have long since disappeared. Successive generations of kids became hooked on reading through John's *The Iron Duke*, *The Duke Decides*, and *The Kid from Tompkinsville*, all still in print today. His autobiography, *A Measure of Independence*, was an absorbing account of growing up poor in Boston where his widowed mother ran a boarding house for students in order to send her two sons through Harvard. The book told of his service overseas during the First World War and of his beginnings as a reporter and novelist. The book went into several printings, and chapters were selected for inclusion in three anthologies. In a long and productive lifetime he published over two thousand magazine articles and three dozen books, most of them for young people, whom he sought to inspire with his own uncompromising code of good manners on the playing fields. In the dog-eat-dog world of book publishing, John was unique: it was his lifelong policy never to ask for or accept an advance on a book. "If the book is worth an advance, it will show up in its sales. I don't want to put money in my pocket for a work not yet completed."

John Tunis graduated cum laude with the class of 1911 and until the end of his days he waged a campaign against any Harvard practices that he deemed elitist. Long before it was commonly accepted, he advocated opening enrollment to women on an equal basis with men. He favored scholarships for minorities and was instrumental in setting up a tutoring program in the Boston area to help disadvantaged youth prepare for Harvard's entrance exams. During the late 1960s and early 1970s he spoke out against the presence of the ROTC on campus and he objected to contractual agreements between industries and the university. During the years of the Vietnam War he added his voice to that of the student body, protesting an American military presence in southeast Asia.

For Jack he was a wise and knowledgeable mentor and did much to point him toward courses that would eventually prepare him for his own successful career in publishing. During World War II when Jack's duties as a pilot in the Army Air Corps kept him in the south Atlantic, North Africa, and Europe, John encouraged him to write about his experiences and then followed up that advice by acting as Jack's agent, submitting Jack's articles to major U.S. and English magazines. The modest income produced by his wartime articles was gratefully accepted by Jack's parents, who were struggling to stay afloat economically in wartime America, as there was scant interest in investing in the printing machinery for which his father was a senior salesman.

After the war Jack was approached by several airlines, as were so many pilots who had been so superbly trained at taxpayers' expense. "And since I really loved flying I probably would have succumbed to their siren songs if it hadn't been for John. But John wouldn't let up until he talked me into going to Columbia's journalism school on the G.I. Bill. Sometimes I think I took that route just to get John off my back."

We often had lunch with John when he would come into New York from his home in Connecticut. He brought to the table all the enthusiasms and energy of a man half his age. But it was an energy unfailingly tempered with a gentle disposition and a self-deprecating wit that lent a new meaning to the word *modest*. He was slight in build and wore the diffidence of a homely man like a comfortable suit of clothes. The deep-set eyes below a brow made extra wide by hair that had receded into near invisibility gave him the look of a sage—thoughtful, even scholarly. But when he laughed the sage became a wag as pleasure lightened his features and rearranged his deep facial grooves into an expression of ineffable delight. It was apparent to even the most casual observer how deeply John relished life. You could hear it in the flat Boston accent that he never lost and see it in his gait, always hurried as if impatient to explore the future. In conversation he was an indefatigable listener. He would sit tilted slightly forward, fixing the speaker with an owl-like gaze, intent on not missing a single word. Everything, his demeanor suggested, was potentially interesting. It was no misimpression. A lifetime as a journalist had endowed him with constantly sweeping radar to alert him to even the most minuscule fragment of newsworthy material. Not much escaped his scrutiny. I often told Jack that John Tunis was the best wedding present anyone could ever have given me.

After John died he remained in our lives, just offstage. How often some incident or other would cause one of us to remark, "Wouldn't John have loved that." Or when faced with an ethical dilemma we would ask, "Well, how would John handle it?"

He was for both of us, even after death, a very real presence.

*

We were well into our second spring. The onset of Jack's Alzheimer's lay eighteen months behind us. Little by little our household had fallen into a sort of rhythm that accommodated his reduced capabilities, his expanded needs, and my inexpert efforts to serve both. Our outdoor forays were shortened. Routines were simplified. A morning visit to the blood lab, an evening drive to watch the sunset, a visit to the orchard country to see the trees bedecked in blossoming finery—one such expedition was all that could be contained in any one day. Jack's speech underwent ups and downs. Usually, but not without a struggle, he would find the words he needed and on those rare occasions when the search was unavailing, I was able to guess what he was struggling to express.

Molly O'Brien had stopped by. As always she came with her clipboard and checkoff list of details pertaining to Jack's condition. This time her visit would be slightly more extended than usual, thanks to additional state-mandated health forms to be filled out. Fine. Was there any reason why I couldn't leave the house for a thirty-minute errand? No reason whatsoever. "Be off with you," Molly told me. "We've been hoping for a little time, just the two of us, haven't we, Jack?"—a bit of blarney that he was quick to acknowledge with a grin and an emphatic "Yes, by all means. We'll be fine, Molly and I."

Upon my return, I saw Molly to the door and then went and joined Jack where he was sitting on the deck, enjoying the end of May sunshine.

"So how are things with Molly?" I asked.

"With Molly?"

"Yes, with Molly."

A fleeting expression of confusion darkened his features and then he brightened and reached for my hand.

"He sent you his best," Jack told me. "He wanted to know what you were up to. He always asks about you."

I hooked my foot around a chair and tugged it closer so I could sit beside him without pulling my hand away. With my free hand I smoothed his hair back from his forehead. He met my gaze with a half smile, an expression of deep-seated satisfaction.

Not ten feet from where we sat a wren was singing a lusty song of proprietorship atop a birdhouse that just a few days before I had hauled out of winter storage and hung in the ginkgo tree. I listened to my own words spoken against a backdrop of birdsong.

"Who sent me his best? Did somebody stop by while Molly was here?"

"Molly? Was she here? I don't think so. No, I was talking to John."

"To John? John who?"

Jack rolled his eyes and tossed his head, a gesture of impatience and annoyance. "John Tunis," he said, speaking clearly and emphatically.

"He was here?" I spoke my words with extra care, setting them out very slowly, one by one. Jack's gaze wandered briefly over the tiny wren, its throat swollen with unsung notes, and then he turned his head and seemed to search my features.

"John said . . ." he faltered, lost the thread and then in a few seconds found it again. "He said it was fine. He said he liked it a lot."

I sat very still. The wren's call, lusty, defiant, triumphant, swelled in the grass-scented air. We sat together, Jack and I, my hand in his. With great deliberation, I took one huge, wobbly breath to pull the wren's song inside my head. And there, for several merciful moments, it blotted out all reason.

*

In Peter Shaffer's haunting play, *Equus*, the psychiatrist, Martin Dysart is entrusted with the treatment of a disturbed boy who blinded a stableful of horses by stabbing their eyes out with a knife. The play is based on a true story that took place somewhere in rural England. It received wide press coverage at the time. I remember Jack's reading the story in the Sunday newspaper and calling my attention to it. There was something gruesomely fascinating about an act so bizarre, so inexplicable, so horrible. We spoke of it several times afterward, musing out loud about what on earth could have possessed anyone to do this.

Shaffer must have had much the same reaction. But whereas we read the article, were horrified, and went right on with our lives, Shaffer pondered the same account and from it fashioned the play that held audiences enthralled on both sides of the Atlantic. In the play's final scene, Martin Dysart, in a hauntingly moving monologue, speaks of how he will relieve the boy of his illusions, the illusions that caused him to blind the horses. But in doing so he will also forever end the boy's conviction that the horses were divine deities with which he alone could communicate.

The world in which we live seems, decade by decade, to be stripping itself clean of illusion. Children, even quite young children, are being handed books that deal with issues that only a generation ago were reserved for adulthood. Do eight-year-olds really need to be reading stories about drug dealers, incest, and spousal abuse? About parents sentenced to jail for crimes they did or maybe didn't commit? Aesop and Mother Goose, Pinocchio and Babar seem to be increasingly eased out of early childhood by socially correct tales that obviate any need to let the imagination soar. Like Martin Dysart, I can't help but wonder, is the obliteration of illusion necessarily for the best?

If Jack believed that he and his dear friend had spent an afternoon together, well, why not? "Delusional thinking," as every textbook on the subject tells us, is almost invariably a part of Alzheimer's. One article I read suggests "gently guiding the patient back to reality." But why? If the experience was comforting, why not let it be? And even in saying that I recognize that illusion can distress quite as readily as it can delight. Well, I thought, we can deal with that when, or better yet, if, the time ever comes.

17

For 300 years, physicians have speculated about what mystery caused people with dementia to become anxious, agitated and helpless. In 1907, Dr. Alois Alzheimer, a German neurologist, uncovered a clue: cerebral abnormalities. Using a special staining technique, he performed a neurological autopsy on the brain of a 56-year-old woman who had complained in her journal, "I have lost myself." Dr. Alzheimer found accumulations of plaque around nerves and unusual bundles of cells in the cerebral cortex, the part of the brain responsible for memory and reason.

www.nytimes.com/partners/microsites/fromcausetocure/
alzheimers/index.html

So much of who Jack was was shaped by his childhood during the Great Depression. A warm house. Supper on the table at seven. New shoes when school started. None of these were to be taken for granted. They were privileges. In those days, pre-Social Security, pre-Medicare, pre-unemployment insurance, pre-student loans, pre-food stamps, just staying afloat financially and caring for one's family required a mental stamina undistracted by thoughts of IRAs and Keoghs. He grew up in a household where books were borrowed from the public library, not bought in the bookstore. Shirt collars were turned, shoes were resoled. The bounty of the backyard vegetable patch was poured into scalded glass jars and husbanded against the layoffs of winter. World War II brought the curtain crashing down on all of that. But left behind were ingrained habits that even the easy ways of the millennium's last decades couldn't erode.

In our household he was steadfast in his resolve never to buy on credit. No car loans. No borrowing. No indebtedness of any kind. His wallet was full of credit cards, but he used them only with reluctance and the statement was paid before the end of the month.

In a name-brand society he was wonderfully unaware. One make of sneakers, one brand of coffee, one kind of tennis racquet was as good as any other. If the fit, the taste, the feel was tolerable, if the price tag matched the cash in his pocket, fine.

"Just charge it," to the sales clerk were words I doubt he ever spoke. But ask him what brand or what make he'd chosen, and he'd shrug off the question. A typical reply: "I didn't really notice, but it was a pretty good price."

His years as a pilot in the U.S. Army Air Force passed him along into the arms of the G.I. Bill from which came his master's degree from the Columbia School of Journalism. On graduating he quickly landed not one but two jobs. For several years he worked a day shift at one paper, a night shift at another, surviving on four or five hours of sleep. Early retirement was never one of his goals. He worked nonstop to the age of seventy-three.

The big strike at the *Times* was called by the printers' union, over its concerns about automation. The other unions showed solidarity by joining the strike. Jack was a longtime member of the

Newspaper Guild. But even had he not been in the guild, he would not, on principle, have crossed the picket line.

My immediate reaction in the first days of the strike, was, Great! Where can we go! Suddenly this lovely smooth empty expanse of time was laid out in front of us. At my own work I still had unused vacation time. There were bargain-priced fares to everywhere—London, Paris, Rome, Tokyo, Sydney, Rio. A golden opportunity! But it was not that simple.

"When the strike ends," Jack told me, "anyone not back at work within twenty-four hours is automatically dismissed."

"Even if you have plenty of vacation time coming to you?"

"Even then." So much for that.

So it was into this interval, this ill-defined, no-work gap of time that Hagos Legesse materialized. Hagos was one of those mysterious people, flung outward across the world by the chaotic swirlings of revolution. His home was Ethiopia. Exactly what complication, what clashing of ideologies expelled him into exile, we never knew. Did he leave of his own free will? Did he leave just a few steps ahead of some official paper that would have brought him to trial or perhaps face to face with a firing squad? He never said. We never asked. He came to New York like so many others who settled in clumps on the West Side, in Queens, and in New Rochelle. Often there was some vague affiliation with a consulate or the United Nations, with Ox Fam or a foundation. A never clearly defined connection with a faceless somebody, somebody who could pull strings, provide vital introductions, who "knew the ropes." Regardless of education, family background, or professional calling, all of these new arrivals had one bond in common: They were survivors.

I've long since forgotten the name of the restaurant where we met, but fixed forever in my memory (if any memory is forever!) are the details of the meeting.

"He said to bring you, too," Jack told me, as he was shrugging on his overcoat, preparatory to departing for dinner someplace way uptown.

"He? What he? You never said anything about . . ."

"This Ethiopian. Who wants to have dinner with us. It's an Ethiopian restaurant. We're both invited. He was emphatic. Didn't I tell you?"

"I don't think so."

"Well, anyway. Come on."

It was a nasty night. Rain was slapping like wet laundry against the windows of the loft. I had letters to write, calls to make, and a brand new book that I was saving like a child saves candy, deliciously holding off a treat. The choice of staying home versus a long subway ride uptown on a wet night seemed pretty easily made.

But Jack pulled my raincoat from the closet and held it out for me.

"Come on. Even if you don't much want to. It's a long way up there and back. Come keep me company." So of course I went.

The restaurant on Amsterdam Avenue was hard to find. Indoor shutters, closed and latched, prevented any light from its windows falling on the rain-slick pavement. The dark tin numerals of its address were practically invisible, positioned as they were above the black-painted doorway. The name appeared nowhere. Total anonymity.

Hagos Legesse was not my first Ethiopian. That honor was reserved for Haille Selassie, the Emperor of Ethiopia, the King of Judah, the Lion King. Not the Disney creation but the real thing, tracing his royal line back to the time before the pyramids. A diminutive, frail figure of such immense dignity. Displaced. Aged. But still standing as erect as if he were in the flag-draped stands of his homeland, proudly taking the salute of the elephant-mounted royal guard. I remembered his wearing his ceremonial robes, to deliver his plea to the United Nations, a plea that everyone knew was hopeless.

He was my first Ethiopian, known of course only from photographs. And, as it turned out, of not much use in preparing me for my second Ethiopian.

Hagos was there ahead of us, already seated with a couple of waiters buzzing around him like attentive bees. Introductions were exchanged, so sorry to be late, quite all right, so kind of you to come out on a night like this—all muddled together in a swirl of awkward cordiality. In the flutter that went with the removal of our wet coats, I searched but failed to find much of the King of Judah in Hagos Legesse. Just for starters, he was solidly built, in the full prime of middle life. By some odd trick of the dim lighting, his dark eyes shone with unusual brilliance, as if what little light there was pooled in his eyes. When he smiled or laughed, they crinkled into slits of merriment. They were very expressive eyes and as a mirror of his moods, probably, I thought, more reliable than his words. He had a broad, pale-cinnamon face and a luxuriant three-sided black mustache. It was a face not well designed for duplicity or subterfuge. His English came easily, though no one would have mistaken him for native-born. When he spoke to the waiter it was in quick sharp spurts of indecipherable sound.

Jack and I sat side by side on a banquette. Hagos sat across from us in an elaborately carved chair. His one versus our two. An even split. We were no sooner settled than, without our having ordered, dinner began to be served, fragrant steaming platters of food impossible to identify. And palm wine, which I sipped and found so appallingly dreadful that I assumed it was some kind of a mistake. But that notion went by the boards when Hagos, after a few words of welcome, tipped back his glass and drank with unconcealed pleasure.

The French consider it poor form to discuss business before the cheese. Americans, of course, are not bound by any such niceties. Nor are Ethiopians. Hagos didn't wait for the cheese.

Jack's name, he said, had been given him by a friend of his in the State Department, an under-under-secretary for African affairs. He spoke his name and Jack shook his head.

"Never heard of him," he said cheerfully.

No. Of course not. Because that man in the State Department, had in turn been given Jack's name by someone else. And the someone else was indeed a longtime friend of Jack's. A college friend, a tennis friend, a newspaper friend.

With that disclosure, some middle turf of trust materialized between the two. While Hagos spoke, changing shades of unbridled enthusiasm and optimism played across his face like lights from a projector. Novelists write of "contagious enthusiasm." If that expression has any validity, I guess I can say I was seriously infected right from the start.

It seemed that Hagos had a Grand Plan. He wanted to start a magazine on Africa. A bimonthly. He even had a name. *Africa Update*. It would cover political developments, trade, environmental issues, tourism, the arts, culture. Everything! Illustrated of course.

Funding? No problem. He had sources. Up high. And of course such a magazine would be a magnet for all kinds of heavy-duty advertisers because, as he put it so simply, "There's no other U.S. publication on Africa out there. Where else could an advertiser go?" Fees for writers and photographers, well, yes, they'd be modest. "Until we got underway." He already had midtown office space. It should be possible to get the first issue out within the next three months. Content for the first issue? He already had a folderful of ideas. He'd found a printer, out on Long Island. An advertising manager, yes, that was a tough one, but he was already working on it and had one or two possibilities lined up. By the middle of next week he should have that cleared up. He whisked lightly over a few other details and then, finally, laid down his fork, took a long draught of the dreadful palm wine, and sat back to look at us. "So, what do you think?"

Jack nodded emphatically. "I think it's a great idea."

Me, too, I thought, but had the decency to keep it to myself.

"I was sure you would," Hagos beamed. He stretched a hand across the table. "So are we agreed? You'll come along?" He waited to clasp Jack's hand in a promise of . . . well, it wasn't really clear. Partnership? Collaboration? Certainly some kind of agreement.

The hand remained, unmet, lying palm up on the dark batik tablecloth.

"But I don't see," said Jack, "what I have to do with all this. Did I come up here just to listen? To tell you what I thought? Because if so, I can think of any number of people whose opinion on something like this would be of much greater value than mine. I'd be glad to put you in touch with . . ."

The hand moved to take a firm grip on Jack's cuff. Hagos leaned forward with enormous energy. "I've not made myself clear. It's not your opinion I want. It's you. I need you as my editor."

Whatever Jack was thinking when he agreed to this meeting, and maybe he wasn't thinking much of anything beyond dinner uptown in an Ethiopian restaurant with someone who sounded, well, interesting, offbeat, it was immediately clear that hiring on as editor of a nonexistent magazine was way outside his concept of the feasible.

But he took his time. He pushed back his plate. His lifted his glass and drained, without wincing, the rest of the god-awful wine.

He fished his pipe from his pocket, filled it, lit it, and drew in one long, slow, and wholly satisfying lungful. He sat back and surveyed our host who met his gaze with hopes undimmed.

Then, carefully and clearly, Jack went on to explain that yes, he was not working but no, he was not out of work. The strike at the *Times*, no matter how prolonged, would eventually end. Days, weeks, maybe months, though he doubted that. Once it ended, he would again resume his regular editorial duties. He was, in other words, not free to accept this very kind offer.

Of course. All that was understood. But for the moment, until the strike ended, until then, would Jack make himself available?

"Wouldn't you be much better off finding someone who could do the job on a permanent basis?" Certainly a sensible question.

"Nothing is permanent," came the smiling reply. "Is that not so?" this last directed at me. But I had no intention of taking sides so I merely smiled and thoughtfully turned my wine glass in gentle circles, taking care not to spill its brimming contents. "Why can we not make an agreement that is no more than day to day?"

Jack glanced over at me and raised his eyebrows, twin thickets that posed his question as clearly as words. And I, to my everlasting credit, replied demurely, "It's up to you."

Before the evening ended, Hagos turned to me to say, "And I'm sure we could use you, too. I read your piece on Scotland, in the *Washington Post*. Very nice." It was such a neat little bit of flattery. And it proved how thoroughly the groundwork for this meeting had been laid.

For the next several weeks Jack labored full-time in that trio of midtown offices. Three rooms laid out railroad car style. Two small rooms, each with a window, served as bookends to the larger middle room, no window. All pre-computer era, of course. Editorial work was done in the middle room. Awful lighting. Shared desks. Perilous swivel chairs. Second-, probably third-hand, type-writers. Only two phones, both with knotted, tangled lines that came from being handed back and forth. Even the dented waste-baskets must have been salvaged from some former life. It was a crowded, messy, happy space.

As the battlefield is distant from HQ, so was that middle room distant from the publisher's office. Hagos presided from behind a good solid door that was almost always firmly closed. Within all was carpeted and upholstered. His was a handsome mahogany desk, the correspondence of the day, neatly centered behind an imposing pen and pencil set, the kind that is ceremoniously awarded after decades of corporate fidelity. Across the top of his bookcase, aligned in a tidy row, stood small silk flags of newborn African nations. The walls were hung with brightly colored framed posters that trumpeted the comforts of flying Air Afrique, KLM, or Air Gabon. From the window there was a fine view of the up-town skyline, the tops of the tall buildings crocheted together by the contrails of jets zooming in and out of La Guardia.

The third office, directly across from the elevators, was acces-sible through the pebbly glass door, neatly inscribed AFRICA UPDATE, the black letters smartly outlined in gold. A small sit-and-wait area provided a tableful of come-to-Africa brochures and two or three inhospitable plastic chairs. Behind the reception desk you could always count on finding a comely, dark-skinned young woman, soft spoken, efficient, but never there for long. The turn-over was nonstop. A week or two was the norm. As quickly as one vanished, another would take her place. A different name but al-ways the same demeanor, diffident, speaking in such low tones one had to lean forward to catch what was being said. Poised and unruffled, these young women handled phone and visitors with quiet dispatch. They dressed in the bright gauzy sheaths of their distant homeland. As graceful, as fragile as gazelles, they wore circles of gold around one arm, just above the elbow. They wore complicated earrings and interesting bits of shell or shiny stones woven into ebony hair. For a while, during Bokassa's reign, there was a brief succession of young women from the Central African Republic. They spoke an English dipped in French. Knowing what they'd left behind, the crazy emperor with the solid gold bed and the schoolchildren hacked to bits in the Bangui basement, it seemed important to address them as gently as possible. They were creatures of mystery, these receptionists. Often Jack and I marveled but never learned through what pipeline they had traveled from the African continent to that small, stuffy office in midtown New York. And when they departed, where did they go?

The magazine came into existence at a time when all of Africa seemed to be trembling on the brink of enormous change, but change for the better or for the worse was far from clear. In the north, Algeria had won its independence from France a decade and a half before *Africa Update* was born, an independence that came only after seven terrible years of civil war. Karen Blixen's Africa of colonialism under white Europeans was fast disappearing. Most Americans thought of Africa—if they thought of it at all—as safariland. Hemingway in his tent camp. William Holden shouldering his elephant rifle. The great white hunter. Passion in a sleeping bag on the snowy slopes of Kilimanjaro. But investment in Africa? Very low priority.

China and the Soviet Union took a different view of the "dark continent." After Suez, Egypt had asked the U.S. to finance the building of the Aswan Dam. When the U.S. declined, the Soviets happily stepped into the breach to build the dam. Its completion was heralded with lots of kudos for the Soviet way of life. It was not a scenario that our State Department was anxious to see repeated. So proposals for bridges and dams, railways and high-ways, which otherwise would have kindled little enthusiasm in the halls of Congress, received respectful attention because, "If we don't do it, they will."

Names that sat comfortably in Western ears—Northern and Southern Rhodesia, Salisbury, the Congo—easy to spell, easy to pronounce names, were fast being replaced by exotica: Zimbabwe, Zambia, Harare, Zaire. Men and sometimes women, all with strange-sounding names, made public pronouncements in the name of their embattled or newly liberated countries. With increasing frequency African names were cropping up in U.S. newspapers. Jomo Kenyatta, Kenneth Kuanda, Joshua Nkomo, Julius Nyere, Robert Mugabe, voices speaking on behalf of infant nations, more often than not embroiled in fearful bloodletting as power passed from one faction to another.

Jack was hooked. When the strike ended, he returned to the *Times*, and once again he was holding down two jobs. He spent most of his lunch hours at *Africa Update*, and at the end of each day he would bike over again, hang up his jacket and resume work. There I would join him when my own workday was finished. It was not unusual for us to be huddled over inky proofs or typescript until well past midnight.

Jack appealed for help to the dean of Columbia's School of Journalism, who dispatched a succession of student interns. Without exception they were eager, hardworking young men and women, bright, funny, and rotten spellers. They came and went at odd hours. Were they even paid? I can't remember, but my guess is they weren't. They came because none had ever encountered a Hagos Legesse or facsimile thereof. They came because the idea of working up close for an emerging magazine was very seductive. They stayed because working under Jack's direction was an education in itself.

Africa Update covered south of Sahara and north of south, meaning that, with apartheid in full command, South Africa was excluded. But within those parameters Jack preached a policy of all-inclusiveness. "Just ask," Jack would tell a hesitant intern, debating how to approach a Nobel Prize winner living in Cairo or a key speaker at the United Nations. "And when they refuse, ask and ask again."

Requests flew out to congressmen, heads of state, diplomats, political dissidents, CEOs, naturalists, journalists, geologists, sociologists, poets. Anyone who had something of note to contribute about Africa was fair game. The magazine blanketed the whole vast continent with an exuberance born of the absolute absence of competition. Oil exploration in Chad. Saudi investments in Mauritania. Can Dakar's industrial free zone succeed? A close-up of world trade in Africa's endangered species. Air fare deregulation. Civil war in Angola. Rebellion in Mozambique. Cocoa blight in the Ivory Coast. Ivory poaching on the Serengeti. Bird watching in the Seychelles. Hippo nursery in Tsavo West. Walking the Luanga River Valley. It was a heady feeling knowing how inexhaustible the subject matter.

Sometimes Hagos came with us on our trips to Africa. Sometimes I went alone. From each trip we returned with heads and notebooks crammed with impressions of worlds light years away from our own.

Each homebound trip, from Arusha, Dar, Dakar, Nairobi, ended in an interminable overnight flight, often fifteen hours or more. We would find ourselves landing in the small hours at Kennedy. Then came the shuffle-by in passport control, the long wait for our bags to come tumbling down the chute, inspection by customs agents, with occasionally a Very Official Somebody rooting in search of contraband through our dusty, dirty luggage. Weary beyond utterance we would reenter the sleeping city where, once within our own four walls, I would drop into bed hoping for nothing more than an unbroken week of sleep. My return to ordinary life was a slow, uneven process.

Not so Jack. With the first light of day he would be up, showered, dressed, and on his bike, cheerfully pedaling his way up to the *Times*. He appeared to be blessed with an iron constitution that could jet through half a dozen time zones to pick up his regular workload without missing a beat. I don't think I ever heard him speak of jet lag or even simple exhaustion. Having worked hard since the age of fourteen, he was able to return from strenuous forays abroad and, without missing a stride, resume his regular work routine.

It was a talent I envied. I had no gift for the instant turnaround. For a week or more I would semi-sleepwalk the city streets, with the sights, the sounds, and the smells of Africa lingering in some deep chasm of my senses. Biking through the city traffic I would recall clearly and with delight the barefoot busyness of African marketplaces. Tugs and barges plying the rivers around Manhattan evoked the watery traffic between Dar es Salaam and Zanzibar where white-robed Arabs still stalked the streets like their slaver ancestors.

Why, I often wondered, was I, a pale-skinned creature born and bred on the eastern eyelid of North America, so susceptible to Africa, to its smells, its tastes, its sounds, its sights. Had I believed in reincarnation, which I did not, I would have understood that my previous life or lives had unfolded somewhere on that unfathomable continent. How else to explain why so much, experienced for the first time, was totally unsurprising, was even, in some puzzling sense, comfortably familiar? As on an early Zambian morning, stepping out and hearing, not, I was certain, for the first time, that distinctive four-note call of the doves: whoo-WHOO WHOO-whoo-o-o-o. As at midday, when my head would fill with the relentless humming that was the baked-grass chorus of locusts, grasshoppers, crickets, tree frogs, and armies of small winged creatures rustling unseen underfoot and overhead. Even at night the vast roster of animal sounds seemed a fragment of a long ago dream, the grunts, snorts, howls, and dark snuffling noises, the hoot-hooting of night birds, and the high-pitched squeal of a hapless creature in its death agony. And the heady smells of Africa—had I carried them always in some deep cranial crevice, authentic and intact, like microscopic olfactory seeds? The fragrance of wood smoke, sun-cooked earth, charring meat, fermenting fruit. The rich, satisfying dark smell of hair-covered hides and drying dung. Not just déjà vu but déjà heard and smelled and tasted. Somewhere, sometime, I'd been there before.

Of course I knew just how idiotic a concept it was, a concept I was not about to share with anyone, not even Jack, especially not Jack. He was far too even-keeled to traffic in nonsense. But then one afternoon from an unexpected quarter, came what I chose to take as vindication.

We were in Tanzania, leaving the Ngorongoro Crater, headed by doubtful jeep to Arusha, due east of us. But thirty-six miles due west of us was the Olduvai Gorge where the archaeologist/anthropologists Louis and Mary Leakey had spent the better parts of their lives in search of fossilized human remains. Somewhere in the early days of *Africa Update* a folder of correspondence had come into being, the magazine hoping for an article from Louis or Mary Leakey, and the Leakeys hoping for some kind of exposure that would assist in their unending quest for funding. We were pressed for time, with a plane to catch in Arusha that with luck—always a scarce commodity in that part of the world—would get us back to the U.S. in time to return to our "real jobs." But thirty-six miles was irresistibly close. We did not resist.

Mary Leakey apologized for her husband's absence. He was "off beating the bushes for money," which meant a speaking tour in the U.S. "But I can give you an idea of what we're doing here." Her sun-grizzled features were shaded by a shapeless cotton hat that, like her short-sleeved shirt and baggy skirt, had assumed the color of the dusty landscape of rocks, earth, and gorge, all bleached to a mono-chromatic tan. She spoke in terse, clipped phrases that betrayed her English origins, but her eyes beneath the hat brim were clear and bright. We found cordiality, even welcome, not in the tobacco-husky voice but in her gaze, eye to eye and unwavering.

Jack explained how pressed we were for time but told her that the chance to stop by the gorge was too precious to pass up. She nodded emphatically.

"So let's not waste time," she said promptly and turned to lead the way from the car park where we were standing in the unfor-giving sun. She marched ahead of us, a blunt, irreducible figure, purposeful even from the back.

We stood, the three of us, on the edge of a deep cut in the earth gazing down at a handful of workers. Into the distilled hot air Mary Leakey exhaled fragrant clouds of cigar smoke. "If you had more time," she told us, "we could go down and I could show you just how we work here. But since you're on a short tether, let's just step over here and you'll see what it's all about."

We followed her into a kind of lean-to where shelves of un-painted boards were covered with small pieces of dust-colored objects, many no larger than the tip of a little finger. All were in the process of being identified and cataloged. On the floor were hand-woven baskets filled with more such pieces, each marked with a small tag.

Some pieces were bone. Others were tools. Stone Age. All had been recovered from the gorge, which, maybe two million years ago, had followed the shoreline of an alkaline lake. When surrounding volcanic activity obliterated the lake, the creatures that frequented the area were buried with ash and lava.

As she spoke, a slim, barefoot African in shorts and a T-shirt entered the small enclosure and stood deferentially aside, awaiting a break in Mary Leakey's explanations.

Turning abruptly and seeing him standing there, she hastened to introduce us. Dr. Nyerere, she told us. Both Jack and I were caught off guard and our bewilderment didn't pass unnoticed. Smiling, the newcomer shook hands saying in a soft, even melodious voice, "But no relation to President Nyerere," and we all laughed.

He was, we learned, Tanzanian, a Ph.D. anthropology graduate of St. Andrews in Edinburgh. Despite his youthful appearance, he had already chalked up more than twenty years working with the Leakeys at a variety of African sites.

If Jack was interested, Mary Leakey told him, she had a recently updated report on work here at Olduvai. Could he make use of a copy? And when, in accepting, he offered to mail it back, perhaps with a few additional copies, he was treated to a huge smile that bespoke a friendship sealed.

They turned to leave and I said I'd be right along. But I lingered, idly fingering some of the earthen-colored objects spread out, not randomly as I'd mistakenly thought but in some kind of scholarly order quite indiscernible to an untutored eye.

At my elbow Dr. Nyerere lingered, a half smile playing over his features.

"You appear taken. Will you perchance join us here?"

His accent—was I just imagining the faintest Scottish burr?— and his oddly formal word choice disconcerted me for a moment.

"You mean to work? In the dig?"

"We have many volunteers. Quite a few from your country. Some are students, but we also receive people who come for a fortnight, even a year. Though many are quite outside the world of scientific research, they occasionally make very significant contributions."

His gentle tone, his quiet way of speaking, would, I thought, go a long way toward offsetting the relentless heat, the hours of squatting and touching with a brush, as insubstantial as a feather, the dusty, dry, earthen walls of the gorge. It was work for the impassioned, for the Leakeys of the world, for the Dr. Nyereres, too, I supposed. But the time in which to dedicate myself to anything like that had passed me by long, long ago.

No, no, I said dismissively. I just find something about the antiquity of all this, I indicated the cluttered space, well, and I searched for the right word. "Compelling," I said lamely.

"As do we all," he said softly. "Look, over here. Mary didn't show you. She's far too modest, always pointing out her husband's work. But her own finds have been . . ." and it was his turn to search for the right word. "Extraordinary," he finished.

He leaned over and from off a low shelf he withdrew something swathed in layers of soft cotton cloth. With infinite care he folded the layers aside and held out in both hands a plaster mold.

I stared at it, not knowing what I was supposed to see, not grasping its significance. I looked up and waited for an explanation.

It was a plaster cast of half a skull. "It's human?" I asked, laying a tentative finger on its yellowish smooth surface.

"A hominid skull we'd call it. Zinjanthropus."

How old, I asked, and was told 1.8 million years.

It was Mary Leakey's very own find, discovered in 1959, down in the depths of the Olduvai Gorge and hailed throughout the world of anthropology as perhaps the most significant find of its kind in the last century.

"Significant how?" I asked, with the unabashed candor of the ignorant.

Dr. Nyerere laughed a little, gently folding the cloths back into place.

"We each answer that in our own way," he told me.

"Well, how do you answer it?" I pressed him.

"Me? My personal opinion or my scholarly opinion?"

I considered the choice.

"Personal."

He gave me a grin that I could only describe as conspiratorial.

"This was," he lifted the swaddled object as if to offer it to me, "the head of my ancestor. Or, to put it more correctly, a mold of the head of my ancestor."

"And mine as well?"

"Most certainly."

We shared a moment of silence, each of us breathing in the heat of the African midday, the air scented with cigar smoke and dust. I watched him replace the skull, handling it so deliberately with something akin to reverence.

"Our common ancestor," I said.

"Our common ancestor," he repeated, taking my hand in his and shaking it with a certain finality from which, right or wrong, I derived a hugely satisfying sense of vindication.

18

The fog, as Carl Sandburg said, comes on little cat feet. First you notice that you are always misplacing things, or that common nouns are evading you as stubbornly as the names of new acquaintances. Pretty soon you're forgetting appointments and getting flustered in traffic. On bad days you can't hold numbers in your mind long enough to dial the phone.

Geoffrey Cowley, *Newsweek*, January 31, 2000, p. 46

Once we returned home, the images of Africa would gradually recede, the colors fading, the wonderful smells of dust and dung and spice and heat driven out by city fumes. But it was a slow process.

There was, however, one trip from which Jack did not return with his characteristic aplomb. We were in the sauna city of Libreville, the capital of Gabon that straddles the equator on the eastern shores of the south Atlantic. The city was hosting the annual summit meeting of the Organization of African Unity. To house the event, a brand-new convention hall had been built, complete with air conditioning, multilingual translation equipment, elevators, and state-of-the-art press booths. A newly constructed six-lane boulevard led from the city center to this multimillion dollar palace. (Returning two years later we found the structure stripped of its handsome cherry-red seats, its marble washrooms. Pipes, copper tubing, and electrical wires had been surgically excised. Except for tropical growth around it, it could easily have passed for any stripped-down building in Chicago, the Bronx, or Los Angeles.)

Following the summit's adjournment we had a two-day interval before the next flight from Libreville to Paris and thence on to New York. It was an opportunity Jack had no intention of missing. He spent a busy half-day buttonholing the appropriate officials, making the necessary phone calls, and securing the mysterious permits that seemed always to precede any African excursion. Early the next morning, with Derek Anderssen, a Dutch photographer, in tow, the three of us boarded a pint-sized Cessna for the thirty-minute flight from Libreville to Lambourene, the small market town on the Okoume River where, in 1913, Albert Schweitzer had built his famous hospital. Recently the hospital had been in the news following a large-scale upgrading and a general shake-up of staff. Jack wanted to do a photo essay about the hospital in *Africa Update*. On a more personal level, we both had read extensively about Schweitzer's extraordinary life and were curious to visit the outpost to which he had so energetically devoted such a large part of his life.

From the Lambarene airstrip it was a dusty truck ride to the river banks, where a fleet of pirogues waited, as orderly as taxis in a London lineup. Many were heaped high with huge stems of bananas, with piles of coconuts and enormous bundles of sugar cane. Trading was brisk between the buyers along the shore and the farmers whose produce it was. It was a noisy, cheerful scene that unfolded quite heedless of the temperature, which, even well before noon, was easily into the three figures, with the humidity tagging right along behind.

We managed with a minimum of fuss the business of engaging a boat that would take us upstream to the hospital. Our request generated no great flurry of curiosity or interest. A couple of boatmen volunteered and then amiably settled between them which one would take us. We clambered with care into the narrow boat, Jack and I having a considerably easier time of it than Derek, who came laden with a heavy satchel of camera equipment. Traffic was brisk up and down the river, with boatmen and passengers exchanging greetings, often amidst gusts of laughter and cheerfully shouted insults. A sputtering outboard motor, attached to our pirogue by nothing more reliable than a frayed length of hemp rope propelled us slowly up against the current. The fumes of the motor blended with the smell of river water and the hot moisture-laden air. The effect was like intermittent whiffs of a general anesthetic, sleep-inducing, quelling all thought of physical exertion. When I dangled my hand overboard, the river water, flowing through my fingers, was the color of tea, as warm as tea. The landing, when we came to it, was no landing at all. No dock or wharf. Only a brief break in the green wall of vegetation and a few square yards of sand, riven with the keels of other pirogues. From the middle of the river, only an experienced eye would ever have spotted it.

Jack climbed out and extended a hand to help me over the high sides of the boat.

"You OK?" he asked.

"Fine. Just hot." He lifted the hair off the back of my neck and just the micro-instant of air on my damp skin felt wonderful.

We trudged up a brief slope that leveled out beside a small enclosure, hemmed in by a rusty iron fence. The rude stone cross inside the enclosure was almost completely hidden by voracious weeds. The inscription was economical: Schweitzer's name and dates, January 14, 1875–September 4, 1965. The three of us stood there, surveying the sad little plot in silence. I think I had expected something more impressive. Or perhaps it was coming upon it so immediately that threw me off balance. Or was it only the relentless equatorial heat? The vaporous air was a weight on my eyelids that sent salty sweat down my lashes to puddle, stinging, in my eyes.

The gravesite was shaded by a thick canopy of tree limbs from which tough-stemmed vines hung in languid loops as if poised to reclaim it. A brown and black ribby goat with ears as limp as old gloves was browsing along the fence. When I leaned down to pet it, it shoved a hot, wet nose into my palm.

While Derek went about the business of photographing the grave, Jack led the way to a clearing where Monsieur le Directeur sat waiting for us. He was perched in a worn canvas sling chair under a huge ficus tree. He started to rise, but when we hurried forward to shake his hand, he sank back with visible relief.

Doctor Karl, he told us. And, yes, he was expecting us. Our plane, he observed, had landed an hour late. He rather thought we'd be here sooner.

Had word of our arrival sped upstream ahead of us?

Old, I thought. Corn-colored eyebrows jutted out over watery blue eyes sunk into a sun-cured face, dark as a winter apple. I pegged him for mid-sixties. His trousers and long-sleeved shirt were dust-colored cotton, the shirt buttoned high to his throat, the sleeves buttoned too at his wrists. I noted his shoes, thick-soled and ankle high with leather thongs wrapped several times around and firmly tied. Beside him I felt uncomfortably vulnerable, my dusty feet encased in nothing more than the crisscross of thin leather sandals. Should I have given consideration to nameless creatures, snakes, lizards, maybe spiders, that lurked unseen at ground level? But just the sight of his armored feet made me feel the day's heat with even greater intensity.

We sat on wooden benches while he spoke to us in German-accented English, courtesy of his university and medical school training in his native Zurich. He had an almost languid way of speaking with long pauses between thoughts as if the mere effort of putting together a coherent account was wearisome.

His story and the story of Albert Schweitzer's hospital were so intimately interwoven that it was often impossible to tell if he was speaking his own thoughts or passing along those of Schweitzer, his revered mentor.

He wore a battered pith helmet that served him as diversion the way a smoker fingers pipe and pouch. Every few minutes he would doff his hat and swipe a tattered navy blue kerchief around the hat band before jamming it back atop a headful of bristly gray-white hair.

Yes, he had worked closely with Dr. Schweitzer.

"A saint. I know that for a fact." He made the pronouncement emphatically and then paused, looking hard at each of us as if expecting some refutation.

But we hadn't come to debate the merits of the man. We'd come to record in a very modest way some evidence of his life work. He went on to tell us that he had first arrived at Lambarene as a young medical intern in the late 1950s. He described a two-year tour of duty that I took to be something like our own Peace Corps, administered by French officialdom.

"Of course, I knew nothing of tropical diseases. Here, in only six months I saw and learned about maladies that back in Europe are known only in textbooks." That first stint in Lambarene had been followed by several other stays of less than a year until, twelve years ago, he consented to come out as director for a four-year commitment.

"I was promised a replacement after four years." But a replacement was evidently not easily found. The four non-African staff doctors at Lambarene were unsalaried. Indeed, they had to pay their own traveling expenses as well as a monthly stipend to cover room and board.

"It's so difficult, as you can imagine, finding qualified physicians who can give three, two, or even one year of service out here." It seemed like an understatement of considerable proportions. His tour of duty here, he told us, would soon be over. In fact, his replacement should already have arrived, but complications, some government confusion in Libreville, or perhaps not Libreville, perhaps just delays in the shipping schedule—he was coming by boat from Marseilles—something had caused delays. But within a week, maybe two, he would be departing. Yes. For good. After a dozen years as director. Things were changing. It was time he went. The government wanted to see the hospital turned over completely to African personnel, and why not?

"Our time here is finished," he said, not elaborating, and leaving us to invest it with whatever meaning we chose.

Did he mean that the future of the hospital was in doubt? Or was he referring only to a change in personnel that would see an end to whatever remnants of colonialism remained?

We would like, no doubt, to be shown through the hospital, no?

As I listened, I recalculated. Not mid-sixties at all. Closer to his early fifties. Worn down or burned out, but certainly not old.

Jack explained that he hoped to run a photo essay about Lambarene and the work being done there in an upcoming issue of *Africa Update*. Could Derek be given permission to photograph?

Yes, of course, we were told. Then to our surprise he pulled from the outsized pockets of his cotton shirt a couple of severely battered back issues of *Africa Update*, displaying them proudly. "Of course, they arrive quite out of date since they are sent by sea. But you understand, I'm sure, that anything that can be done to remind the world of the hospital's existence, well, it can only be a help."

And so began our tour. He was nothing if not thorough, our guide. He showed us first the old buildings, the ones built under Schweitzer's personal direction. Of concrete, originally covered with thatch, they now were topped with corrugated tin. No electricity. The only light came in through small, slatted windows. The rooms were small and stripped to bare essentials. The laboratory had a single shelf on which stood an antique microscope, an inkwell, a dip pen, and a schoolboy's ruled notebook.

Derek trailed behind us, lingering at each stop to photograph. Jack kept step with Dr. Karl, his head inclined attentively to the pith helmet. From time to time he asked a brief question, but for the most part was satisfied simply to listen to the accounts of what had transpired in these bleak surroundings.

Almost from the moment of our arrival we acquired an entourage of children, wide-eyed and seemingly delighted by our presence. I tried a bit of French on the older ones. They replied, shy, and convulsed in giggles, but nothing they said was intelligible.

"They seldom know French," the doctor told me, pausing to swipe out his hat. "If they go to school, which is rare, they're taught in French. Missionaries usually. But their language is Fang." But I noticed whenever he spoke to anyone, child or adult, he spoke only in French and seemed not to heed or care what he was answered in return.

Almost every child carried a smaller one on his or her back. Some of the bearers could hardly have been more than four, yet they tagged along, toting an even smaller scrap of humanity in a calico sling, knotted over shoulders thin as bird wings.

Every patient admitted to the hospital had to be accompanied by someone who could prepare his food, tend, feed, and administer prescribed medication. Paid nursing was an unknown, and indeed there were only four nurses on staff, working for the most part in surgery and obstetrics.

We were shown Dr. Schweitzer's bedroom, a monastic cell, preserved as reverently as a shrine. The cot was draped with musty mosquito netting. Beside the cot, black high top shoes like a pair of Old Town canoes. A small writing table (could the knees of a large man really fit under there?), an old-fashioned ink well, dip pens with rusty nibs, a gold pocket watch and chain, and a mildewed pith helmet hanging on the wall—that was all. In the equally small room adjacent to where he slept stood the upright piano, presented to the great man by the Paris Bach Society, in recognition of Schweitzer's accomplishments in preserving dozens of pipe organs all over Europe, priceless treasures that, had it not been for his protests, would have been discarded to be replaced by inferior modern instruments.

Finally we were led to the new clinic. It was placed on a ridge, overlooking the river and stood in wondrous contrast to all that came before. The floors and walls were of easily scrubbed, shiny white tile. Double roofs were suspended above the walls to allow for the free circulation of air. We were shown the operating room and consulting rooms, and glimpsed modern-looking X-ray and dental equipment. Most of the equipment had been donated, primarily by French and American companies. By Western standards it was all pretty basic, but when viewed in the context of what had been, it could be considered nothing less than miraculous.

The smell of cooking fires drifted in the glass-free windows. We could hear high-pitched children's voices, ragged with laughter and punctuated with abrupt maternal phrases that needed no translation. We were led through a long, low hut, roofed in thatch where patients lay, some on cots but many stretched on lengths of cloth laid on the earthen floor.

Jack asked what was the most common disorder, a question that seemed to catch the doctor by surprise. He paused, staring thoughtfully at his heavy shoes. He stood, motionless, while he considered the question. After a long moment he began.

"Tuberculosis," he raised both hands, ticking off each entry on outspread fingers. "Syphilis, cholera, schistosomiasis, poliomyelitis, typhus, pneumonia, tetanus, hepatitis, cryptosporidium." There were no fingers left. "And leprosy."

Jack started to say something but the doctor hadn't finished. "That, of course, does not include the subordinates."

The subordinates?

He nodded and then, in the face of our obvious incomprehension, he explained with the patience of a conscientious teacher, "Yes. There's malnutrition, of course, as well as snake bite, hippo attack, crocodile, hyena, even lion, although, come to think of it, we've not seen lion attack for quite some time, six months, I'd say. And we deal fairly regularly with amputations—hands, arms, legs—that sort of thing."

The amputations were easy to spot. An arm, a leg, encased in bulky bandages, the victim, sitting or lying expressionless, watching us pass without interest.

I mentioned that I saw few children. Why was that?

Children, he told us, were traditionally treated in the village by the village doctor. "They have their own methods, you know. Some of them surprisingly effective. But more often than not, infection sets in and then it's too late to make the journey here. Measles, too, is very prevalent. Here in Gabon, measles is deadly."

We ate lunch in a small house, one of the few where windows were covered with netting. Two other physicians, one from Boston, the other from Montreal, joined us, as did a cheerful young woman, a native of Florence, who was completing a survey for the World Health Organization. All would depart before the year ended.

A thick, cold bean soup, a plate of sardines, and a bowl of sweetened yogurt completed the meal. Cold bottles of beer were placed on the table, and when someone noticed that I passed on the beer, a small flurry ensued and I was brought a cold can of an orange drink, so sweet it made my teeth ache. Derek ran off his last roll of film. It was time to leave.

We headed single file for the landing, the doctor leading the way. Heat, fatigue, and an unshakable melancholia gripped me. I felt an urgent need for silence and solitude, time in which to assimilate the sights, sounds, and smells of the day. Maybe Jack felt as I did, for he was exceptionally quiet as we wended our way toward the river.

He was walking just ahead of me. Suddenly, he stopped. I had to hop aside to avoid bumping into him. I opened my mouth to speak but his upraised hand stopped me. We were just passing a small house of whitewashed slats. It stood off the ground on foothigh pilings. No windows. The door was locked with a hasp secured by a stout peg.

A tool shed. Some sort of utility outbuilding. But as we stood there we could hear distinctly human sounds, something between weeping and moaning, seeping through the horizontal slats. We took a step closer to see a long row of eyes peering out from between the slats. Five, six, maybe eight pairs of eyes, wide, dark, intensely focused eyes, stripped of gender and age.

Ahead of us Dr. Karl paused, and turned back. The sounds rose to an eerie wail and then subsided. He met our gaze and nodded as if to acknowledge our bewilderment. "It's the best we can do," he explained. "Without sufficient medication, all we can do is keep them safe in there where they can harm no one, including themselves." He used the French word: *les foux*. The crazies. We stood transfixed, our eyes locked onto those other eyes. It was as if we were staring back into the absolute depths of anguished humanity.

Our pirogue was waiting. Our departure was brief. The trip downstream took only half as long as the trip upstream, and we had no trouble getting a ride back to the airstrip. There was some delay concerning the return plane to Libreville, and the three of us, Derek, Jack, and I, sought refuge from the afternoon sun on a bench in the shade of the little administration building. We sat in silence, each lost in our own thoughts. At last the plane arrived. In ragtag fashion we gathered ourselves together to cross the tarmac, Derek first and I tagging along behind. I'd taken but a few steps when I realized Jack was not with us. I turned back.

He sat slumped, his clasped hands between his knees, his head bowed, the very picture of desolation. I touched his shoulder. "It's time," I said gently. "The plane." After a moment he looked up. He stood then and shouldered his knapsack. We walked together to the waiting plane. He didn't speak. When we reached the small ladder of the plane, I tossed my own knapsack in. As I started up the steps, I looked over my shoulder. Jack stood directly behind me wearing an anguished expression that bespoke more than the heat and fatigue of a long day.

"What?" I said.

"Those eyes," he said, in little more than a whisper. He shook his head. "I can't get them out of my mind." He handed up his knapsack, waited one long moment holding onto the ladder and then he clambered up and took his seat. All the way back to Libreville he sat staring out the window, saying not a word.

19

One worker showed how Alzheimer's patients in the early stage of disease pass through a period during which they become excruciatingly aware of their memory loss. As their memories continue to deteriorate, they become less cognizant of their loss.

John Horgan, *The Undiscovered Mind*, p. 234, Free Press, 1999

It was June, about seven months since Jack was stricken. He had regained much of his mobility. His speech was, usually but not always, intelligible. He tired very easily and names eluded him, but his improvement since the onset of the illness heartened me. We awoke after not too restless a night to birdsong and brilliant sunshine. I turned over carefully. He was lying beside me, so still that I was sure he was still asleep. His eyes were wide open but a despairing expression filled the hollows of his face.

"What is it?" I asked in something that sounded more like a whisper than a voice.

"Just a dream," he told me. "That's all. It was just a dream." But he made no motion to rouse himself, to shake off the dark shadows that lingered on from sleep into wakefulness.

I waited but he continued to lie there, wide awake, the pillow bunched up under his cheek, unable or perhaps unwilling to free himself from whatever images that held him prisoner.

"Do you remember the dream?"

"Of course," he said, with an emphasis that struck me as odd. For me, indeed I rather think for everyone, dreams are as elusive as cobwebs that once broken can never be glimpsed again in their wispy totality.

"So tell me."

He closed his eyes for a long moment and when he reopened them he began to speak clearly, without hesitation, as if he were describing a scene that he pictured in absolute clarity.

"I saw myself standing there. In darkness. Inside the small house, I was staring out through the boards and I saw you there, on the outside, looking straight at me. But you didn't recognize me. I called to you. But everyone else inside the house was calling, too. Calling and crying out. You didn't answer. You saw me. I know. But soon you turned and walked away. So I was left there. With the others."

"The others? Who were the others?"

"Don't you know?"

"If I knew, I wouldn't ask you."

"The crazies."

So then, of course, I did remember, and once remembering, wondered how I could ever have forgotten. Some thirty years had passed since that long equatorial day in Gabon. On that perfect morning in June that faraway scene—its sounds and smells, its terrible legacy of human suffering and sorrow—flooded back with startling clarity.

I reached over and folded Jack's hand into mine and for several minutes neither of us spoke. I had to wait for the morning to reassert itself, for the gift of sunshine and our togetherness to rescue me from that long ago darkness. But the now, stronger than the then, won through and finally I was able to speak with reason and common sense.

"It was only a dream. That's all. What we saw that day, it probably doesn't even exist today. You read all the time about medications that are used to treat the mentally disturbed. Even over there."

He fixed his eyes on my face, studying it as if he would commit it to memory.

"No. When I stood there, I knew it was exactly right. I felt it then." A pause. "I feel it now."

He thrust back the covers and stood up, ready finally to confront the day.

I sat up too, watching him cross the room, the nightmare's horror replaced by the sanity of daylight, home, the safety of the moment. But in the doorway he turned.

"Who believes in prophecies? Not me and not you either. But that day in that godforsaken place, those people, the crazies as the doctor called them, you can't convince me it wasn't prophetic. All of them in that lock-up shack, they'd lost their minds, every one of them. Just the way I'm losing mine."

A rush of water. The slam of the shower door. And then, sitting there in the rumpled bed, I recalled a childhood saying, a legacy no doubt from my southern-born father: Don't tell your dream before breakfast unless you want it to come true.

20

In the study, scientists inserted human tau genes into mice which later developed masses of abnormal tau filaments in nerve cells within the spinal cord, cortex and brainstem, three critical regions of the central nervous system. As the mice aged, insoluble masses of tau filaments grew in number. The animals also showed evidence of nerve cell degeneration and impaired movement, unlike their littermates lacking the inserted tau gene.

National Institute on Aging News: Alzheimer's Disease
Research Update, November 23, 1999,
www.alzheimers.org/nianews/nianews24.html

"It isn't clear that animals use the same kind of memories that humans do," said Dr. Pearlman, whose company is delivering several memory enhancers. "A mouse doesn't have to remember a PIN number to get along during the day."

Interview with Dr. Rodney Pearlman, president and
chief executive of Saegis Pharmaceuticals, conducted by
David Tuller, *New York Times*, July 29, 2003,
Section F, p. 6

Theories abound, and I don't doubt that before the mystery is finally solved, many ideas that today are receiving respectful attention will end up on the trash pile of medical speculation. But because I find it easier to confront something of which I have a reasonably clear picture, I have formulated my own theory. I visualize the brain, that three-pound chunk of soft, pink, wet meat, as a coral reef across which algae are growing, just the way I've seen algae smothering the reefs off Key West, off the Great Barrier Reef, and down off the San Blas Islands. The algae creep and spread and flourish, smothering life out of the coral, turning living cells into dead, white lifeless stone. It's not, I grant you, a theory that would stand a chance in the labs or classrooms of any respectable medical institution. But until something better comes along, it's the visual picture that I held in my mind when trying to imagine what day by day was happening to Jack.

Despite the formidable amounts of energy that the infant *Africa Update* claimed, as a rival to Jack's affections, it never even came close to the *New York Times*. For it was from his work as head of the paper's book publishing division that he derived the most satisfaction. The division was conceived as a means by which material researched and written for the daily paper could be further developed into book form. Over the years dozens of such books were published on topics that ranged from man's first exploration of the moon to Craig Claiborne's recipes. It was the very nature of such a book publishing program that the pipeline never ran dry. There was always another civil war, another environmental disaster, another military coup in the Third World, and who knew the details more intimately than the hard-working men and women who staffed the far-flung bureaus of the *New York Times*. Jack's enthusiasm for the program, his unstinting support for the writers and his meticulous editing skills were responsible for persuading many a reluctant reporter to undertake the massive amounts of work required to expand newspaper articles into book form. It was work in which he totally immersed himself, and in the process crafted friendships with men and women of wonderfully diverse interests. Our household operated on a revolving door system that brought a constant flow of overnight and weekend guests, passing through New York with half-completed manuscripts and a powerful reluctance to pay the price of a midtown hotel. For them Jack was more than a gifted editor. He was also friend, advocate, promoter, and tireless enthusiast. He believed absolutely in their abilities, and when publishing schedules required his devoting entire weekends to readying a manuscript for the printers, he gave himself over to the task without a murmur of protest.

21

Imagine your brain as a house filled with lights. Now imagine someone turning off those lights one by one. That's what Alzheimer's disease does. It turns off the lights so that the flow of ideas, emotions and memories from one room to the next slows and eventually ceases.

Adeline Nash, *Time Magazine*, July 17, 2000, p. 51

Why did we return again and again for "evaluation"? Common sense told us loud and clear that "out there" was nothing of any use to us. No magic pill, no surgical intervention, no physical therapy whereby what was lost could be recovered. Still, every few months, there we would be, Jack, relaxed, compliant, unconcerned as to the findings.

He sits comfortably on the examining table, indifferent to the blood pressure cuff, the perfunctory checking of neck glands. As always, Dr. X is professionally cheerful and no less unconcerned. And why should he not be? He is not about to stumble across any dramatic syndrome on which he could base a paper to read at the next wholly tax-deductible medical get-together in Fort Lauderdale or Santa Fe. He is not about to be challenged to come up with a proper medication, selected from a menu that offers conflicting choices, all based on incomplete data.

And I am at liberty to study the treetops outside the window or the artwork that seems to change from one visit to the next. Who selects the art for offices such as this? Surely not Dr. X himself. No, I think, given the maniacal organization by which the medical industry is administered, chances are there is a company, and highly profitable too, devoted to the sole purpose of providing appropriate artwork to offices just like this. It's easy to imagine the parameters. Biblical scenes are out. Natural disasters—flood, tidal wave, earthquake, volcanic eruptions—are out. Poverty, Dickensian or otherwise, in all its colorful phases of starvation, homelessness, hypothermia, child and spousal abuse—all out. War, no but military parades are maybe. Bucolic landscapes, woodland scenes, seascapes—can't get enough. Fire is out, although possibly the Great Fire of London, 1666, makes it through. Misty lake scenes, all those views of the Cotswolds—acceptable, except perhaps in offices where asthmatics are treated. Wordsworth's mists could too easily be misconstrued as particulates, formerly known as just dirty air.

This time my eye passes over and then returns to the reproduction of a picture I remember well. The original hangs in Albi. No need to approach it to read the initials in the lower left corner.

It's a painting of a horse, not a sleek, steeplechasing horse, just a plain horse, a gray barnyard horse, doubtless as accustomed to traces and harness as to saddle and bridle. He has a barrel for a midsection—no oats for him, just grass or hay. The horse is galloping away from me at an angle, hooves churning up the dust along a weedy country path. There's a young boy in the saddle. The boy seems dressed in ordinary farm clothes. No boots or spurs. No cap or crop. Though I can't see his face, I know with absolute certainty that it's split wide in a grin. Running behind the horse and quite a distance behind—I doubt that he'll catch up—is a little dog. He is to dogs what that horse is to horses. Ordinary and nothing special. No collar. No weekly grooming or flea powders. Like the boy in the saddle, the dog, too, looks happy, racing along behind his good friend, the horse. It's a picture vibrant with motion. The horse, the boy, the dog, running, racing for the sheer muscular joy of it. For the sensation of air rushing through nostrils and thundering on eardrums. Drying spit in the mouth and parting hair right down to bone and skin.

And is there, I wonder, any correlation between the painting and the fact that the artist, that dwarfish, bristly French aristocrat, could never experience for himself those same heady sensations, confined as he was for life to foreshortened legs that made even standing so painful? Musing on that point, it's not much of a stretch to wonder if the same correlation exists between this picture on this wall and the patient for whose enjoyment it hangs there, the patient, who like the artist, is unlikely ever to know, in whatever time remains, the animal pleasures of racing full speed ahead.

Dr. X, having accepted today's version of the clock, the wobbly circle with the numbers inscribed, I don't even want to know where, now moves on to the rest of what I've learned is called the "7 minute screen."

He enunciates very clearly. First he says the four words slowly but without pausing: Tunnel. Apple. Mr. Johnson. Charity. He asks Jack to repeat each word after him:

Tunnel.
Tunnel.
Apple.
Apple.
Mr. Johnson.
Mr. Johnson.
Charity.
Charity.

"Now in five minutes, I will ask you to repeat those same four words. Alright?" Jack nods, looks over at me with a half smile, a smile that asks, What are we doing here and how soon can we leave?

The five minutes pass with flashcards of fruits and vegetables, and never mind that browsing the produce section of the market, or even browsing the market itself, was never Jack's specialty. Orange. Lemon. But kale? Broccoli? Onion? To be fair, that onion could easily pass as a turnip, but then he wouldn't know turnip either. Not now. Not twenty years ago. Strawberry. Good! Mushroom, no dice. Finally we return to that all-significant quartet of words. Of the four, Jack recalls tunnel. Mr. Johnson, charity, and the apple have vanished. Well, I think to myself, tunnel is probably the most sensible one to hang onto. Tunnel. It fits both of us very nicely.

22

What is the 7 Minute Screen?

The 7 Minute Screen is a screening tool to help identify patients who should be screened for Alzheimer's disease. The screening tool is highly sensitive to the early signs of AD, using a series of questions to assess different types of intellectual functionality.

It can distinguish between cognitive changes due to the normal aging process and cognitive deficits due to dementia, of which AD is the most common form.

Janssen Pharmaceutica Research Foundations
and AMA Procedural Terminology, 1994

Alzheimer's. The forgetting disease. The gradual but eventually complete erosion of memory. Deprived of memory, who are we? Can we continue to love those whose names escape us, whose faces no longer even look familiar? Whenever I tried to think myself inside Jack's existence, to imagine the mental landscape where he was living, I met head on with defeat. I couldn't manage.

Sometimes, as if in refutation, I'd mentally construct the anti-Alzheimer world: Supposing our brain, idiopathically assaulted, misfired in the opposite direction? Supposing instead of duly noting and then discarding life's nonessentials, our brain retained it all? Not tidily tucked away in the storeroom of memory, but right up front in our daily consciousness. Every scrap of trivia, every phone number, zip code, street address, every musical passage (casually whistled, sublimely executed), the detritus of the morning papers, the entire play, the 150-minute film—its dialogue, sets, sound track—all retained. Every reply, comment, exhortation, wisecrack, heard or overheard, every public announcement or private confidence. Every odor, fragrance, stink, every visual image, every flush of terror, delight, ecstasy, all boredom, all apprehension, all sense of pain or well-being, every word lifted from the printed page—all locked on-screen, not in some unvisited fissure of our brains but in a pink, steadily pulsing, perfectly nourished frontal lobe. Vivid and immediate, right there in the forecourt of our brain.

How devastating such a mental disorder! But then, was it really any more implausible than what was happening to Jack? And if indeed my imaginary anomaly were ever to be realized, ghastly as it might be, would it be one whit less devastating than loss of the brain's ability to provide us with the context of a voice, a face, the touch of a hand? With the context of love? Would it be any less devastating than Alzheimer's?

It was the photograph in a magazine advertisement that caught my eye—two figures, two women, old and young. The old in oversized glasses, pink plastic pearls to match the pink cotton sweater, facial features, well into the sinking seventies but for this one instant, hoisted upward into the semblance of an almost-smile. She stands, half a head shorter than the young, the optimistically thirty-year-old, sunshine beaming through a headful of blond curly hair, a casually buttoned blue shirt and a smile that holds nothing back. She lays a protective arm around the shoulders of her mother? aunt? grandmother?—a picture that clearly bespeaks a bridging of the generations. Youth safeguarding Age. Youth extending concern and care and maybe even affection for a needy someone. And above the picture in large upper-case type those seventeen letters that now circumscribe our lives: ALZHEIMER'S DISEASE.

So, of course, I read the accompanying text. It was all laid out in scrupulously chosen phrases, phrases that would certainly prove impervious to any lawsuits that might ever be mounted by the opportunistic, the stricken, or the merely adventurous. Clinical trials were taking place, it said, all across the country. Invited to participate were people aged 52 to 85, "in the early or middle stages of the disease." I read on. "A center near you is investigating a device-based treatment for Alzheimer's disease. Participants will be reimbursed for reasonable travel expenses."

A *device*? I tried but not for the life of me could I envision what sort of a mechanical device could reverse or alleviate what was happening to Jack's brain. With curiosity but no conviction, I tore the picture out and shoved it into a pocket, intending, well, probably nothing. But a week or maybe two weeks later I pulled on a jacket and discovered the folded page. Well, after all, what was there to lose?

So I called. Maybe if I had investigated further, I might have come to a different conclusion. But I doubt it. It was a West Coast company whose literature announced the successful sale of preferred stock that raised $30 million. From this comfortably secure base, clinical trials would proceed nationwide for which volunteers were being sought. Hence the ad that had caught my eye. The trials involved subjecting acceptable volunteers to surgery under a general anesthetic for the purpose of implanting a "flow-controlled shunt designed to increase flow of cerebrospinal fluid and improve clearance of potential neurotoxins from the fluid bathing the brain." Ah-hah! The device. I read on. It was to be implanted directly into the brain, attached to a catheter that would drain "about 3 ounces of fluid" daily into the abdomen.

Because it was clinical study, there would have to be two groups: one group receiving the implant, the other group not receiving the implant. Both groups, however, would undergo the surgery, although no participant would be told whether the implant had or had not taken place.

Did I wish to receive a tape that would provide further information? I declined with thanks, and after carefully hanging up the phone, I tore the brightly colored advertisement into very small pieces and dropped them safely in the wastepaper basket.

23

The [7 Minute] Screen may be administered by a nurse, physician's assistant or other support personnel. Only minimal training is needed, and no preparation is required.

The average amount of time required to conduct and score the screen is 7 minutes, 42 seconds.

During the screen, the patient is seated opposite the administrator.

After the administrator provides a brief explanation of the 7 Minute Screen, the testing begins.

The 7 Minute Screen consists of four separate tests, each measuring a different aspect of cognition (intellectual functioning) that is typically compromised in persons with Alzheimer's disease.

Janssen Pharmaceutica Research Foundations and
AMA Current Procedural Terminology, 1994

Then came the time when our fragile craft, too hastily designed, sloshing and tipping in the turbulent seas of illness, began to shift alarmingly. Like it or not, I was being edged overboard by a rival.

And what a seductive temptress she was, shoving ever more greedily between us.

Sleep.

She hovered at Jack's elbow, never quitting, never giving up.

As soon as breakfast was over: "I think I'll just go lie down for a while."

Or, saying nothing, sitting by the window on a fine day with the whole world waiting just beyond the glass, Jack's head would nod, his eyes would flutter closed, and he'd be gone. Sleep was my rival and the struggle to defeat her was never ending. She was forever luring him out and away from whatever scheme I'd devised to keep his muscles working, his mind, or what was then passing for his mind, up and running.

"Come walk with me to the mailbox. I just want to get these two letters in before the mailman comes." And what difference if the mailman had already come and gone? What difference if this was the third time in one day that I'd used this same feeble ploy?

I lost the battle more often than I won. If I left him alone for only the few moments it took to prepare lunch, to attend to the laundry or tidy the kitchen, he would grope to our bed and fall at once into deep sleep. I plotted all sorts of ways to muffle the siren call of sleep. A ride in the car was often my best, my only bet. In the first week or so after Jack was stricken, I had taken our two cars, his and mine, back to the dealer. Both cars were middle aged but reasonably healthy. In their place I drove home a second-hand navy blue van, sturdy, reliable, not given to unseemly displays of temperament. Its selling point was the wide door on the passenger side that greatly facilitated climbing in and out.

"See! I melted the other two cars down to make this one. Isn't it great!" This stupid joke was for the grandchildren, repeated far too often but invariably received with appreciative giggles.

"Shall we take a drive? Not long. Just to see how high, how low, the tide is. Just to see if the water is up over the road. Just to see if any of the beach washed away last night, if many branches fell in the storm, if the bridge has reopened, if the nets are up, if the courts are dry." Any pretext sufficed. And invariably, shouldering past his seductress, he would quicken and to my delight, agree that, yes, he'd like to come along. To the post office. The market. Up to the twin lights for a good view of the harbor.

The one-car-out-of-two permitted me to maneuver Jack unaided. Moving cautiously and very slowly. Hold wide the door. "Now turn around and face me. Good, good. Now just sit down. See! Sit back. You're safe." And then sometimes, without, but more often with, my help, his long legs would get folded up, safely placed in front, the seat belt pulled around, and there! wasn't that a cinch! And off we would go, headed . . . did it really matter where?

From behind the wheel I made a valiant effort to keep him with me.

"How clear the light is there on the pond."

"Shall we go up to Mark's house to return Sarah's plate? To drop off this book? To pick up your gloves?"

"Look, look, there's that beautiful, stupid African goose, the one we put in the pond last summer. He must live over here now at the elementary school. I guess the kids throw him their sandwich crusts so he doesn't really need a brain."

For the first few moments he would stay there with me. The sunlight cascading through the windshield would animate his face. Glimmers of who he was would flicker across his features, his eyes open wide to receive the passing world. But in the few seconds it would take me to make a left turn, to attend to a school bus stopping just ahead, my rival would slip in between us and steal him away.

One week folded so seamlessly into another that I hardly noticed the degrees by which our life together was diminishing. When he left the dinner table, his plate hardly touched, I forgot that up until the previous week, he'd enjoyed his food. The next evening I would give him less, and soon the less would become the norm. When he walked only halfway to the road and then, defeated, turned back toward the house, I thought, well, this once but tomorrow we'll do better. The gentle, undeniable decline continued until, suddenly, magically, it was abruptly halted.

24

How Do I Bill for the 7 Minute Screen?

Visits in which the Screen is administered should be billed using code 99214. Because the 7 Minute Screen involves an extensive test administered by your trained staff, the office visit lasts longer than the typical 15 minutes of a visit that would be coded as 99213. . . .

Often, an office visit is billed using code 99213. This visit can normally be described as one with the evaluation and management of an established patient, which requires at least two of these three key components:

- *A problem focused history*
- *A problem focused examination, and*
- *Medical decision making of low complexity*

Jenny arrived.

I never had to wonder where Jenny fitted into Jack's life. Jenny, who had so cleverly contrived to have the same January 20 birthday as her dad. In Jack's life Jenny was the spring of delight that never ran dry. Along the bumpy road from infancy to adulthood, surely there must have been moments when his paternal expectations were not quite fulfilled. Times when some loving word, some gentle gesture on his part went unheeded. Of course there were. But when? None that I ever saw. None of which he ever spoke. Was her approval of her father as wholehearted as his of her? Of that I can't be sure. But I never doubted the strength of their father–daughter relationship.

Marriage, a husband, an infant son, Jack's namesake, had swept Jenny to the opposite side of the country. Instead of weekend visits and phone calls every other day, there was only distance and lots of it. Half a year had passed since Jack had fallen ill and now, with spring in full blossom, Jenny returned, alone, to see her father.

Deliberately I wait until the morning of her arrival, not wanting to tell him lest some unexpected complication pop up that would disrupt her plans. So it is without preamble that she walks unannounced into the living room to embrace him. For the first time in weeks I see him stand up, not painfully or awkwardly but just stand up, as good as ever. He folds her into him and holds on for dear life. When she steps back to survey him I see his face transformed, as if lit from within.

"I had no idea," he tells us, looking from one to the other. "No idea," shaking his head in surprise and delight. "And look how well you are!" And of course she does look well, rosy and healthy, her curly light hair swept back into a luxuriant ponytail, her eyes bright with undisguised affection. But it is his face, not hers, that holds me. It is as if a handful of years have been wiped away, his features once again so alive and expressive, his smile so broad and uncontrived. He puts his arm around her shoulders, not for support but in a protective, loving gesture that is so exactly the Jack that used to be. He tips his head to hers asking for details of what she's been up to. They move out to the deck and make themselves comfortable in the sunshine. I bring tea and we three sit there, legs outstretched, breathing in the pleasures of simply being. They take brief walks together from which Jack returns, weary but contented. His step again is firm. His shoulders that for so long have been bent by the terrible dead weight of exhaustion, are lifted. He holds his head up, the better to keep this much-loved daughter in his sights. She holds his hand and speaks to him gently but with animation. She tells him about her new son, her husband, about her life on the opposite side of the continent. He nods attentively, drinking in the sight of her along with her words. Now and then he asks a question or makes a comment, as if to reassure us that, yes, I'm here, I'm with you.

Dinner that night is a festive affair. He comes to the table, unbidden and erect. He shakes out his napkin and peers across the white peony blossoms at me, at Jenny, with such a natural expression of satisfaction and pleasure that I totally forgive myself for thinking maybe . . . maybe.

Before she leaves I pose father and daughter in front of a scraggly lilac bush that, despite my efforts to encourage it, never amounted to much. But within the frame of the picture, caught in the background, is a profusion of purple blooms. No one looking at the picture would guess how stubbornly unproductive that bush was. In the picture, Jenny, Jack, and the purple lilacs, look so exactly right, so fulfilled and unblemished.

25

An extended visit is billed using code 99214. This visit involves the evaluation and management of an established patient which requires at least two of these three key components:

- *A detailed history*
- *A detailed examination*
- *Medical decision making of moderate complexity*

Is the 7 Minute Screen appropriate to be used with patients from differing cultural and ethnic backgrounds? What about patients who do not speak English as their native language?

The test has been standardized using patients who are native English speakers. If English is not the patient's first language, treat the results with caution.

In my family birthdays were always a big deal. Presents. The children's usually hidden under a chair or high on a shelf. Hunting for them was half the fun. Present-giving for the grown-ups came after the cake, the song, the blowing of the candles. It didn't matter if the present was only a paperback or a holiday T-shirt, it had to be handed over complete with paper, ribbon, and the waste-of-money card.

In Jack's family birthdays, though observed, never amounted to very much. Why wrap the book when the paper's only going to be torn right off? Frugality.

We disagreed on very little. But we disagreed on birthdays.

Mine was in mid-September. It was ten or maybe fifteen years ago. We were treating ourselves to a mid-September weekend on Cape Cod. It had been a just-right holiday with good friends, good tennis, and good weather. Dusk was just turning to dark. It must have been unseasonably warm because we were reclining, our backs against a sand dune. Beach towels over our bare legs to keep mosquitoes at bay. Our bathing suits were dry and stiff with salt. My head rested easily on his shoulder and his arm around me half muffled the not-so-far-off sound of the surf. The air was still ripe with the smell of sun-baked sand, lingering on even into the evening. We both were luxuriating in that special calm that follows a long afternoon emptied of everything but sea and sun. Lying there, side by side, we were peering up into an unblemished sky, so clear I knew we were gazing straight through to infinity.

"Look straight up," Jack told me. "Into that big patch of emptiness. See, right there overhead."

I did.

"Now pick one spot and stare at it as hard as you can."

And I did.

"And just watch. Are you staring hard enough? Don't move your eyes."

A moment or two and then, at the exact point where I was looking, a star, hesitant at first and then clearly distinct, came into view.

"Do you see! You pulled a star out, didn't you!"

"I did! But how did you know?"

"Because I know. It's a trick, making a star appear like that. My Dad taught me that." I tried again, and again the tiny miracle.

"So how do you explain it?" I was trying again in another patch of blue-black sky.

"Willpower. What else."

Then he told me about the night he was flying back to Ascension Island during the war, almost out of gas. "I knew we were on course. I never had to worry about that because I had the world's greatest navigator. Nino Perta. The best. Never off by an eyelash. But the gauge said empty and there was nothing out there but black. I thought, this is it. This time for sure we're headed for the drink and what a stupid way to die.

"Then Nino yells in my ear, 'Pull up those lights, goddammit! Pull them up!' I guess he'd heard me joking around about willing the stars into visibility. But, do you know, that's exactly what I did. I just stared straight ahead, pulling for dear life, because it was for dear life. And what do you know! Those damn lights came up, way out there but dead ahead. And we made it gliding in on bone dry empty."

A thick layer of silence sifted over us, closed in around us. I tried to think about the story. I tried to imagine teetering like that on the brink of oblivion. But I couldn't. The now was too much with me. I closed my eyes against the stars. "That's a great story," I said finally.

"You liked it?" His arm pulled me in a fraction closer.

"M-mm. I did."
"Good. Now it's yours. Happy Birthday."

Another September. Another clear sky. Hale Bopp had come and gone. But blurry pictures of its transit in the Southern Hemisphere still turned up now and then in the science pages of the newspaper. Jack's illness had imposed its own custom-made brand of isolation, gradually walling us off from the rest of the world. One by one we had crossed off the places we could go for dinner. Too many steps. Too much noise. Too long a wait.

Month by month our options for a night out had dwindled. Only one or two remained. Waterfront joints, a cut, but only a small cut, above what we called "greasy spoons." Even in the parking lot you'd pull in a good lungful of fried air before even stepping from the car. Coors or Budweiser or Miller Lite blinked red and blue neon welcomes. From the handicapped parking space next to the wharf, I knew how to bypass the front door, the bar, and the dining room. I knew how to push through not much of a gate to where the outdoor tables perched on the wharf's edge, round tin tables, wobbly, slightly rusty with a hole in the middle for the noonday umbrella.

Not what you'd call elegant. But for us, for Jack and me, it was close to a gala. No need for menus. Chicken in a basket, good for eating with your fingers, that's what worked best. Whatever bits fell to the planking would be cleaned up by gulls before our car was even backed out and headed home.

On the river, fishing boats headed out, running lights lit. Pleasure boats nosed upstream, taking it easy in the No Wake! waters. We ate contentedly, picking at tasteless, deep fried morsels, the coleslaw, the mealy french fries. From out in the dark, voices. Laughing, cranky, officious, or beer-blurry voices.

"No, no, not there, the *other* cleat."

"That was the last one, there ain't no more."

"Not as if I hadn't said."

"If we'd stayed in the bay like he tole us."

"Din I tell you!"

Conversations, fragmented by a fitful breeze and the throb of outboards, floated back to us, looping us into some other existence beyond the limited one in which we now lived. It was pleasant, being included that way, as though we were participants through no efforts of our own. With every passing week Jack was finding it harder and harder to locate and seize the words he wanted, he who had always insisted on word precision. Often I could see that he found the right word, that he had it right there in the front of his mind. But in the effort to move it from mind to mouth, it would slide away and he'd be left, mouth empty, his face contorted with frustration.

I'm seven, maybe eight. In a penny arcade I stand on tiptoe, tense with effort. I press a sweaty coin into the slot and shove home the coin receiver. Inside the glass box lights blink, glinting and gleaming off a dazzling array of small toys. Cheery, hopeful music peals out from somewhere deep inside the machine. A chrome crane comes to life. I clutch the knobs at chin level to maneuver the crane to a coveted toy, a small penknife encased in shiny mother of pearl. So beautiful! I knew just how it would feel in my fingers, that wonderfully smooth, flawless surface. I knew how, dropped into my pocket, a small secret weight, it would confer a kind of private entitlement that was of my own making and therefore so much more precious than any reward from the hands of a grown-up. The jaws descend. They clasp the penknife. They start to swing back to drop it in a channel that would send it sliding down to a dusty aperture somewhere around my knees. But just an instant before the release, it slips from the chrome jaws. It falls back and the crane continues on, stupidly opening empty jaws above the channel.

By ice cream time the stars, by threes and sixes and fours were blinking from off to on. The Big Dipper, about the only constellation I could ever count on finding, had taken shape. Across the dimming sky I drew the imaginary line up to the North Star. I pointed it out to Jack. He looked up, following my outstretched hand. He nodded and repeated, North Star. I wanted to joke, to remind him how once he could pull stars out of the void, could make the invisible turn into light. But I let the thought slide away. Too much effort. Day by day I was getting better at living wholly in the moment, freeing myself of both the past and the future. I was like a traveler with lost luggage, managing perfectly well with just the clothes on my back.

We lingered a bit until the river's chill suggested home and bed. We were just pushing through the rickety gate when Jack turned back for another look at the North Star. "Your birthday, right?" he said. And I laughed. "Today? No, next week I guess."

But I had misunderstood.

"Not the day," he said, a quick flash of impatience in his voice. "The star. Isn't that your birthday? Up there?" And he raised his hand, pointing into the north.

"You're right, of course. I completely forgot."

"So Happy Birthday," and he bent and kissed me somewhere on the top of my head.

26

Is the outcome of the 7 Minute Screen affected by the patient's age, gender, or level of education?

Neither age, gender, nor education has a significant effect on the 7 Minute Screen. . . .

What if I lose the pen? Can any pen be used?

Only pens with dry erase ink can be used. You can obtain replacements at office supply stores."

Janssen Pharmaceutica Research Foundations and
AMA Current Procedural Terminology, 1994

October. Russet, gold, and apple-scented. At noon the sky is too blue to be true.

At night the air is heavy with the promise of frost. The easy cadences of summer seem eons past. It's as if time now has speeded up and the earth is rolling faster and faster downhill, intent on reaching winter's wasteland with all deliberate speed.

The other day I heard that in a single year the earth travels 500 million miles around the sun. Well, it's been just one year since that last blue and gold October. I consider the fact that together, Jack and I have traveled 500 million miles. And I think yes indeed. That sounds just about exactly right.

*

It was a neatly typed letter from a faraway niece. It was full of love and caring and heartfelt compassion for what had befallen Jack: "I only just heard that Jack's been diagnosed with Alzheimer's. What sad, sad news." Her own father had been similarly stricken and had lived out his final years in a nursing home, unable to recognize his only daughter, unaware of his surroundings, unaware of his illness. It was a good letter. I read it over several times before laying it aside on my desk. I would answer it later, in a quiet moment, probably a midnight moment.

That afternoon I coaxed Jack to come for a drive. In this our second autumn I found myself both trying harder and trying less. Was it myself I was seeking to reassure or was it my stricken husband who day by day was drifting further away from the man who was. It was unseasonably warm, a leftover summer day inexplicably shuffled into November. I drove slowly north and west along a narrow neck of sand and bayberry, past wind-warped holly trees and exuberant, jungle-y stands of poison ivy, all the shiny summer leaves now a brilliant scarlet. We lived along the Atlantic flyway. During the spring and fall migrations, bird-watchers by the score turned up, binoculars at the ready, their pockets bulging with *Petersen's Guide* and well thumbed-over checklists. Unexpectedly we came upon a newly constructed boardwalk, courtesy, no doubt, of the parks department. It extended from the sandy road out across wetlands along the fringes of the bay, just right for sighting ospreys, egrets, and southbound cranes. In the far distance a cyclist was receding, pedaling between two dogs, racing along in a delirium of freedom. In a pearl-gray sky the sun, a child's orange balloon, hung an hour or so above the horizon, warding off the chill that night would bring.

I pulled over to the roadside and cut the engine. I intended only to pause a bit, breathing in the day's end, soaking up the serenity that like a mist hung over the landscape of sand, salt-stunted shrubbery, and the bay beyond. In one of those rare moments of self-awareness that come to us all, and vanish as quickly as they come, I thought with a sense of wonder, how profoundly the past twelve months had reshaped me. Waiting, waiting for anything, was something I never managed with grace. It was why I was so often late, foolishly certain that I could always wedge just one more task into a sliver of time—one hastily written letter, one quick phone call, some domestic chore, mindless but essential— and always hurry, hurry or you'll be late. And then, of course, I was late. Yet here I was, on this autumn afternoon, quite content to sit side by side with Jack, empty-minded, oddly at peace. Idly I wondered, where was that other me?

For a moment or two Jack shared the quiet. It was a companionable moment—two people in comfortable harmony. And then, unexpectedly he turned and spoke with a quiet deliberation that belonged to a self I'd almost, but not quite, forgotten. His voice was firm and sure. The gaze with which he held me was as commanding as hands laid on my shoulders.

"We have to speak," he said.

It was not a tone to be met with a wisecrack or a quip.

"Fine," I told him, carefully matching his solemnity. "Can we speak right here?" He considered the question and then shook his head. "Why don't we explore that boardwalk up there. It's new, isn't it?"

My amazement at his tone and at his initiating even so mild an exertion was edged if not with apprehension, then at least with a wariness, a heightened sense of caution. But edged as well with pleasure. Normalcy or even just an imitation of normalcy was oh so welcome.

We got out of the car and hand in hand we made our way to the newly constructed boardwalk. Its boards were still lumberyard yellow. The fragrance of the wood hung pleasingly in the air, quite distinct from all the marshy, salty smells around us. It was built just wide enough for two people, with reassuring handrails along each edge. At intervals benches had been built on overhangs, a design that favored mothers with strollers, leg-weary bird-watchers, and people like us, people whose needs were not quite so easily pigeon-holed.

He walked pretty well, not hurrying but placing each step firmly. He kept his hand on the railing, but used it more as a guide than a support. We were two people on a mission, that much I understood. The fact that the mission was clear to Jack but not at all to me in no way diminished the purposefulness of our journey. Something of his preoccupation conveyed itself to me. We didn't speak, and for once I was content to await whatever fulfillment the day would bring.

The boardwalk meandered in gentle curves, extending maybe the length of a football field. Below our feet and all around us the marsh teemed with the mysterious busyness of the amphibian kingdom. Dragonflies, left over from summer, caught shimmers of light in their wings as they darted like darning needles from reed to reed. In tiny open rivulets, flotillas of waterbugs skittered to and fro in fine imitation of subway rush hours. Canvasbacks fed lazily among the aquatic grasses, oblivious to the onset of the hunting season, only a handful of days in the offing. The boardwalk ended in a flourish, an expanded rounded platform rimmed with comfortable seating space.

"Here," Jack said. "This is fine. Let's sit down here." He was moving and speaking so like his vanished self that reflexively I responded just as I would have five, ten, or twenty years earlier.

"Now look at me," he said.

I turned to face him, the palms of my hands and the backs of my legs grateful for the faint noonday warmth that lingered in the unpainted boards. From behind me the lowering sun lit his face with an end-of-day ruddy light. For an instant I was almost convinced by the healthy glow that bathed his features. He looked so fit, so self-possessed. I caught my breath. This was the face, this was the moment. My thoughts spiraled up and out of reach: Don't move! Don't speak! Just wait here together, you and I. No tomorrow. No next week. Just this. It's enough. I'll ask no more. One finger that gently halts the ticking pendulum of time. That's all.

But then he spoke.

"That letter. Is that letter true?"

"Letter?"

"From Kitty. Is it true? Do I have Alzheimer's?"

"Alzheimer's?" The word, so menacing, so hideous, hung there in the evening air between us. The huge *A* like an insurmountable mountain. The ugly *z* and *h* followed by so unlovely a nasal syllable. And all of it ending in a serpent's hiss. Just the sound of it left a bitter aftertaste in the back of my throat.

"Well, do I?"

"Have Alzheimer's?"

"Yes. That's what I said."

The season in which to ask that question had long since come and gone. Why had he not asked it during our long housebound winter? Or else last spring? Why not during the summer and early fall just passed? Why now? Back then I was prepared. Repeatedly I had rehearsed a few choice phrases, soothing, ambiguous, crafted with care so as not to alarm. They were words to be spoken on a need-to-know basis. But with the passing of time the words had slipped away, lost in the minutia that composed each day of our new existence. How often had I read that one of the characteristics of the disease is the unawareness it confers on its victims. Thirteen months had passed since the dreaded diagnosis was first pronounced, not to Jack lying in that hospital bed, the bars pulled up, but to me, standing in the too bright corridor outside his room.

"What's wrong with me?" Such a simple and totally natural question that anyone would ask, anyone except an Alzheimer's patient. He had never asked it.

"Is that what the letter said?"

"You read it. It was open. Lying there on your desk."

It was not the moment for self-reproach. Such unforgivable carelessness to have left the letter lying there in full view. And never mind that Jack had not been able to read a book or a paper for weeks and weeks. All of that could be dealt with later, in solitude, through faceless hours of the night when I could review, in endless exercises of exquisite masochism, every aspect of my inexcusable laxity.

But that was not for now.

My eyes strayed to the horizon, where sky and water met, not in clear delineation but in a misty band. Maybe if we sat here long enough I could discern the line of demarcation. I wanted to try, wanted to keep my gazed fixed way off there, a safe remove from the small wooden bench on which we sat.

But no. With infinite gentleness Jack reached up, and laid a finger on my chin and turned my head. His gaze was unwavering and fully cognizant.

"Just tell me," he said.

So I said Yes. Just Yes.

It was such a quiet, reasonable dialogue. It belonged to the lives we'd vacated more than a year before. His voice held steady, very low but very steady. He nodded, his features suffused with the effort to hold his thoughts on course.

We waited a bit. What more was there to say? In the end it was his own uncompromising honesty that framed my answer. The white lie, the self-serving half truth, the kind of mild obfuscation to which we all resort when circumstances corner us in awkward moments—that never was Jack. Though I never heard him give the "honesty is the best policy" parental advice to the kids, never heard him criticize duplicity in someone else, the fact was that undiluted candor was as integral a part of who he was as the color of his eyes, the agility of his mind. To have answered his question with anything less than the absolute truth would have been to deny the very essence of who he was.

The light slid out of the sky and at once a chilly wind came up, a timely reminder that this, after all, was mid-November. In mid-November people no longer sit around out-of-doors in the evening light. It was time to go.

I stirred and would have risen but Jack laid a firm hand on my arm.

"But what about you? Are you all right?"

"I'm fine."

"And can we . . . can we . . ." he hesitated, searching. "Can we manage?" he asked.

I wrapped my arms around his neck and laid my head against the warmth of his skin. "We can manage," I told him but the words came out muffled. He didn't hear me. He held me away from him and asked again, "Can we manage?"

"You bet," I said. I kissed him, stood up and held out my hand to help him to his feet. He took my hand, tucked it into his pocket and we walked back to the car in silence. When we reached the house, it was already dark. For just a moment we stayed there in the car, not moving. I reached for the door handle and as I swung the door open, Jack said, "Well, I thought so. But I wasn't sure."

27

No actor ever forgets a role, so I should have realized something was wrong. It was late in 1993 and we were having dinner with my father. We were discussing a 1950s film he made, "Prisoners of War." Finally he looked at me and said, "Mermie, I have no recollection of making that movie."

Maureen Reagan, *Newsweek*, January 31, 2000, p. 55

My carelessness in having left that letter in full view, reprehensible as that was, did not distress me nearly as much as my failure to see or maybe just to guess the extent of Jack's insight. Because he'd never spoken of his condition, I had assumed he was unaware of what was happening to him. Nor was my distress mitigated by the undoubted fact that his insight was transient. In fact that November evening was the only time he ever revealed concern about his condition. It was as if the mists that day by day were thickening over his mind, had momentarily lifted, the way storm clouds can briefly separate, allowing quick, sharp shafts of sunlight to pass across the landscape. But had there been other times when Jack had wrestled with the horrors of his illness, confronting in the privacy of his thoughts the inevitability of losing his mind? Was I naive in thinking that had he endured such moments, I would surely have known? Would have recognized by no more than a glance the anguish of such awareness and been quick to offer loving solace? It was a sobering consideration, a humbling recognition of my limitations.

*

It was a dreary December day. It was a day starved for light, shuffled in between the flamboyance of autumn and the serenity of the season's first snowfall. A cold drizzle had fallen all night and though it hadn't increased, it showed no signs of letting up. A succession of niggling domestic woes had marked the hours from sunrise to mid-afternoon: a plumbing problem in the kitchen that exceeded my plumbing skills. A flipped circuit breaker—but which one?—that made the lights inoperable in half the house. A phone call from Borough Hall advising that our quarterly taxes were overdue. Unless our check was in hand by day's end we would be "in a penalty phase." A grandchild in New England called to report a cutback in Pell grants. Could we advance a four-figure sum, to be repaid by work next summer? Otherwise he would have to drop out for the term. A steady dripping from the dining room ceiling strongly suggested that the patch on the roof was not holding. Some time the night before Jeff had gone a few rounds with a skunk and until I could recall whether he should be bathed in milk or tomato juice, he had to be incarcerated in the garage. From time to time his doleful protests reminded me that we were almost out of milk and had no tomato juice at all. As the day wore on I could feel a scratchy throat settling in, act one, scene one of a head cold that I knew would keep me company for a week.

About three o'clock came a call from the blood lab where we were regulars at two-week intervals. A lilting south-of-the-border voice asked if Mr. Stewart could please come in that afternoon. The doctor had just gone over the lab readouts of the previous day and wanted the tests repeated.

Could it wait until the following day?

Unfortunately not. The lab was closing for a long weekend but would be open today until four. Could we get there by quarter of?

"No problem," I said and felt just the tiniest ping of disappointment when she didn't laugh at my joke.

Jack had lain down after lunch to nap. When I hurried in to explain the situation, I found him sitting on the edge of the bed in his stocking feet. Otherwise he was completely dressed.

Great, I thought. Only the shoes.

I retrieved both shoes and put them on the floor, side by side in front of him.

"If you can just slip these on," I said, "I'll be right back. I have to tie Jeff up outside so we can take the car out of the garage." A hasty kiss and I was off, shrugging my coat on as I went. What should have taken two minutes took five because I couldn't find the chain with which to fasten Jeff to a tree. On the return route I paused just long enough to wash some of the skunk odor off my hands and then headed for the bedroom, grabbing Jack's coat up as I went. We could still make it, I told myself. Just.

I found Jack lying down under the covers, half undressed. He'd removed his sweater, shirt, and socks. His eyes were closed. His shoes were just where I'd placed them five minutes before.

Interested, curious as to how matters would unfold, I stood in the doorway. I watched me rush forward, watched anger and a terrible impatience come pouring out of my mouth. I stood there rooted and saw, with mounting horror how I seized the quilt, threw it back and reached down to pull Jack up, to tug and haul in an effort to bring him to a sitting position. My hands flew left and right. The shirt snatched up, one arm limp and heavy and then the other roughly thrust through the limp sleeves. The buttons, mismatched were being jammed through the buttonholes. The sweater was hauled unceremoniously over Jack's head, not carefully or gently but with sharp, jerking motions. I saw me kneel and reach to shove first one foot and then the other into the shoes and all the while a terrible torrent of words was spewing out of my mouth.

"Don't you ever think of anyone besides yourself? Do you think you're the only one who wants to lie here sleeping the day away? Just to put on your shoes, was that too much to ask? Yes of course it was, and why should you trouble yourself when I'm here to do it for you. Do you ever stop to think that I can get worn out? Does that ever occur to you?"

On and on it went. Not just the words, all knotted and hideous but the shrill voice, like the rasp of saw teeth, edged with an ugly sobbing sound. Stunned, I stood there, watching, listening, appalled by the banality, by the cruelty, by the senselessness of the scene. I was both performer and audience, frozen, helpless to choke off the black and bitter words. The shoes were on his feet. The moment had come to help Jack up so the journey across the room could begin. But as I reached for his hands I saw him throw them up as if to shield his face. It was a gesture of such absolute vulnerability, a mute appeal to be spared the mindless rage that was breaking over him, that was filling my ears and pumping bitter bile into my throat.

It was that motion, the way he raised his hands as if in anticipation of being struck, that shocked me back to sanity. I sat back on the floor, weak with horror. I could feel trickles of icy sweat running down my ribs. I took Jack's hands and used them to wipe the tears from my face.

"I'm so sorry. Please. So sorry. I didn't mean any of it. Just say you forgive me." Remorse poured out in unintelligible phrases. From the edge of the bed he looked down at me, an expression of gentle bemusement on his face. Who was I? Who were we? Some storm had just swept over us but now it had passed and with it the memory of how it had arisen or why. The effort to recall was too much. It was gone and all that was left was this moment, devoid of meaning. With a gesture that was both gentle and exhausted he reached out a hand to help me up. I climbed up onto the bed and lay down like a child beside him. He gathered me in and told me not to worry, it was all right, was, was, sh-h-h-h, sh-h-h-h. And just like that we both fell asleep, our arms around each other.

28

The major aspects of disrupted communications arising in Alzheimer's disease are language problems that result from cognitive decline. One of the first problems to occur involves the forgetting of appropriate words. There is also difficulty naming objects, particularly specific names. The communication problem is not one of articulation but a deficit in generating the appropriate words with which to convey information on a symbolic level.

R. L. Dippel and J. Thomas Hutton, editors, *Caring for the Alzheimer Patient*, 3rd Edition, Prometheus Books, 1996

Glimpses.

The first time it happened I was caught by surprise. It made me burst out laughing. We were sitting in the living room, speaking of, I can't remember what. Trivia of some sort. We had just returned from a brief walk and he was resting, not saying much while I prattled on when, abruptly, he interrupted.

"I think," he said solemnly, "you and I should get married."

I stopped in mid-sentence and stared at him, unsure if he was joking, although joking, like so many other of his attributes, had all but faded from the scene.

When I didn't at once reply, he said it again, this time his voice edged if not exactly with worry, at least with audible urgency.

Caught unawares, I replied as if in fun.

"Do you think we know each other well enough?" I teased. "After all, we don't want to rush into anything, do we?"

It was a fine answer for life as it existed way back when. It was the wrong answer for life as it existed now.

He bypassed my feeble humor and went on, his face etched with the effort to hold his thoughts on a steady course.

"I think we should get married. That's what I want. Wouldn't you like that? Being my wife?"

"I think it would be lovely," I told him, an answer that made him smile and tip his head back, eyes closed, just so quickly sliding into sleep.

That was the first time.

The next time he brought it up, our getting married, I took it more seriously.

"Look," extending my left hand for his inspection. "See that? That's my wedding ring. Let me show you." I slid it off my finger and tilted it to capture the light on the inside of the band. Our initials and the date were etched there in tidy script.

I spelled them out.

"That's us. You and me. And that's the date we were married."

He took the ring from me, fumbled his glasses onto his nose and frowned at the inscription. After a moment he handed it back but there was no satisfaction in his expression. I slid the ring back onto my finger and no more was said.

We were living in the land of impermanence. What was urgent last week was forgotten this week. Our lives were held together by a just one strand of consistency—Jack's downward progression toward oblivion. So I was caught unprepared by his dogged and repeated return to the subject of our marriage. For a month or more he brought it up almost daily. Nothing I could say put his mind at ease.

One day when once again he brought the subject up, and looked genuinely distressed by what he took for my intransigence, I unearthed and placed in his hands our marriage certificate. He held it with both hands, his reading glasses in place, but after a moment or two, he shook his head and handed the paper back to me.

"Shall I read it?"

He nodded.

It was a masterpiece of brevity, a document that dealt exclusively with details required by law, minus embellishments. I skimmed it aloud: name of bridegroom, age, date of birth, occupation; name of bride, age, date of birth, occupation; date of issue of license, county of issue. "I hereby certify that the above named persons were by me united in marriage . . ."

He listened intently.

"And that's us? You and me?"

"That's us alright."

It was an exchange that brought back in vivid detail the afternoon a week before we were married when we paid a courtesy call on one Mason McGinness who would officiate over the proceedings. He was a diminutive man, wiry, brief, with eyes as bright as lasers. He had a manner about him that totally and effectively precluded conversational clutter. Our mission was understood. We were adults. Each of us had been married before. To have so rearranged our lives as to find ourselves now in his study he took as proof positive that this was not a marriage into which we were casually embarking.

"So I take it you both know what you're doing, right?"

Yes, that was right. There were some papers to sign, a few details to set straight, and we would have parted forthwith, the business for which we had come, decently concluded. But somewhere in the minor bustle of affixing our names in the right place on the proper forms, either Jack or Mason McGinniss made some casual reference, although I can't imagine quite how or why, to an event of national import: the publishing of the Pentagon Papers. It would be hard or even impossible to find a subject of greater remove from the business at hand than the dustup that attended the pros and cons of those papers being brought out in book form. But once mention was made, an instant bond sprang up between the two men. The Beacon Press, the publishing arm of the Unitarian Church, and the book division of the *New York Times* were, apart from the Congressional Record, the only two entities that, in defiance of dire warnings from the White House, had nonetheless published the papers in book form.

At once the details of our impending marriage were smothered by an animated discussion of the merits, the perils, the consequences of such publishing temerity.

"We could have been shut down, you know that, don't you?" Mason McGinniss looked positively gleeful.

"I know, I know. No one knew for sure how it would play out."

The whole business could have ended up in the Supreme Court and both publishing houses could have been indicted on criminal charges. The full power of the Justice Department was going to be brought to bear. The two men beheld each other with undisguised pleasure at having stumbled, quite by accident, onto something in which both had been so deeply embroiled. Back and forth they went, swapping delighted impressions and recollections of that stormy chapter of our nation's history. A visit that required no more than twenty minutes spun out to more than an hour with mugs of tea for all of us. Even after all those years, I could still close my eyes and recall how the atmosphere in that small book-lined study positively crackled with electrical energy.

Now, I handed the paper back to Jack and pointed out the signature at the bottom of the page. "Mason F. McGinniss," I read. "Does that name ring a bell?" and even as I said it, I reproached myself. What purpose was served by my calling attention to the ever-widening gulf between Jack and the world around him?

"He married us," I prompted. "Do you remember? We both liked him so much."

Jack studied the signature for a moment before looking up, a question forming in his eyes.

"He married us? You're sure?"

"Sure I'm sure. That's what that paper is all about. It's our marriage certificate."

Jack closed his eyes, laying the paper carefully on his lap. I stretched out my hand to retrieve it but just as I was about to take it from him he opened his eyes and caught my wrist with a good firm hold.

"Mason McGinniss," he said. "You know he was involved in all that business of publishing the Pentagon Papers. Did I ever tell you that?"

But of our marriage, he had no recollection whatsoever.

Glimpses: We were managing. Day by day, by carefully placing one foot just ahead of the other, by not looking left or right and never, of course, up ahead, we were managing. Much of what I'd been told or what I'd read about Alzheimer's was passing us by. Anger, striking out, foul language—not for us. Days of vanished phrases and garbled speech were illuminated by moments of levity that flashed through like summer lightning. Once, during the faceless hours sometime after midnight, I was prowling our bedroom and seeing his arm uncovered I bent over him and tugged the covers higher. His eyes opened. He grinned. "You know, if you were sick and if I was taking care of you, I don't think I could do as good a job."

"Well, that's for sure," I told him, kissing him on the cheek.

I started to straighten up but he held me, my head lowered to his.

"You know," he murmured, "you said that too fast."

Glimpses.

A quiet Sunday afternoon. I was idly leafing through the *New York Times Magazine*, wandering back toward the crossword puzzle. I turned a page and then in a delayed reaction, turned it back. A full page devoted to helping the reader determine whether she or he was headed down the road to Alzheimer's. To facilitate the investigation the author was providing ten warning signs. If you experienced any five of the ten you could well be on your way and you were urged to "see your doctor." I read on.

1. A persistent sad, anxious, or "empty" mood or excessive crying
2. Reduced appetite and weight loss or increased appetite and weight gain
3. Persistent headache, digestive disorders, or chronic pain
4. Irritability, restlessness
5. Decreased energy, fatigue
6. Feelings of guilt, worthlessness, helplessness, hopelessness, pessimism
7. Sleeping too much or too little, early morning waking

8. Loss of interest or pleasure in activities, including sex
9. Difficulty concentrating, remembering, or making decisions
10. Thoughts of death or suicide or suicide attempts

Except for the suicide bits, I had to nod an emphatic Yes. I had all of them. And what, I mused, was I supposed to conclude from that?

Glimpses.

As a working editor Jack was fast and unerring. Line editing and proofreading, page after page, requires a brand of concentration with which I was not blessed. I'm fine for a few pages, for half an hour; but much beyond that, my attention wanders and even my own name, misspelled, could easily float right by me undetected. Not so Jack. He could spot the typo on page 200 as unerringly as the typo on page one. Whenever time permitted I would pass along to him whatever article or review I had completed so he could read it over before I shipped it off. In our house there was no shortage of dictionaries. They floated onto our shelves as review copies, discards from our kids' end-of-term dumpings, all the only-one-buck bargains that neither Jack nor I could resist at garage sales and flea markets. In addition to the usual—*Webster's New Unabridged, Merriman Collegiate*, the Random House, and the two-volume *Oxford English Dictionary* with the magnifying glass invariably missing from the small drawer in the dark blue slipcase, we had the *Reverse Dictionary*, the *Harper's Dictionary of Modern Thought*, plenty of tattered paperback dictionaries in English-Spanish, English-French, English-German, the *Dictionary of Latin Phrases*, and *How To Say It in 25 Languages*. Always, just over the horizon, lay our oft-repeated intention to donate most of them to our local library. But for my own particular needs, I usually bypassed all of them in favor of simply asking Jack to provide me the correct spelling—two l's and one s or two ss's and one l ? So much simpler than looking it up. Jack was my "handy household device." But once the Alzheimer's set in, that convenience too was laid aside. Of course I missed it, but, all things being relative, I saw it for what it was—a very minor matter, far outweighed by more pressing concerns.

It was at the end of a morning, a morning into which I'd crowded an excess of chores. Of top priority was a trip to the post office to mail off a 1,200-word article dealing with the early colonial governments of New England. I had wanted to slip it into the mail before lunch but bad timing now dictated my having to put it off until after lunch. Before leaving my desk and heading for the kitchen I slid the pages into the preaddressed envelope. I was just about to seal the envelope when, on impulse, I took the pages into the living room where Jack was sitting by the window. The morning paper, unread, lay on his lap. His face, empty of expression was turned toward the marsh and the river beyond. At the sound of my voice he turned, something akin to surprise flitting across his features.

I held the several pages out to him and said, as if even nowadays it was the most commonplace of requests, "Would you mind checking these over? You know how bad I am at finding my own mistakes. There's no rush. Just so I get them in the mail before the post office closes."

He took the pages and nodded. I leaned over, kissed him, and lifted his reading glasses, fitting them into place. "I'm going to fix lunch," I told him.

I left the room and while I busied myself heating soup and fixing sandwiches I thought briefly that perhaps I should have desisted. Asking him to read those pages, just as I'd always asked him for so many years gone by, could it end up just depressing him?

Instead of giving him pleasure, was I only reminding him of life the way it used to be? Reminding him of powers lost and lost for good.

It wasn't until late afternoon that I remembered the unfulfilled chore of getting to the post office before closing time. The day was clear. Jack could come too, our outing for the day. Hurriedly I searched the closet for his jacket and cap, gave a quick check along the route he would take to the car, making sure nothing lay in his path that could bring him crashing to the ground. There was my own wallet to find, plus the envelope I'd addressed before lunch, and there was Jeff making ever so clear his hopes of joining the excursion. One of the hardest adjustments I'd had to make to accommodate myself to Jack's illness was simply slowing down. Too many activities jammed into too little time, it was a lifelong failing, seemingly impervious to my once-in-a-while efforts at reform. But now reform was elevated from nicety to necessity. Trying to hurry Jack through any of his day was inviting disaster. Whether it was his washing, his dressing or eating, his walking with me to the car, the mailbox, or just a short ways down our lane, trying to hurry him was totally ineffectual. His fingers would fumble. An expression of bewildered dismay would cloud his features. His gait, already so uncertain would come to a halt as his hands groped for the doorframe, the table's edge or the chair back to steady himself. Over and over again, seeing his distress, I'd admonish myself to slow down! Wasn't there enough to cope with in a single day without my compounding matters with my infernal need to hurryhurryhurry?

So this time I went gently to help Jack into his jacket, explaining that we were off to the post office, Jeff too. I flipped the tweed cap onto his head and took him by the hand. We proceeded carefully from the bedroom, through the living room, pausing just long enough for me to retrieve the paper-clipped pages I had handed Jack before lunch.

"So how were they?" I asked lightly. "Any horrendous errors?" We continued our slow advance toward the back door, the garage, and the car. The business of easing Jack into the car, of fishing for and fastening the seat belt around him, of closing the door, ever alert to an errant foot or finger, absorbed my full attention. I ushered Jeff into the back seat, circled the car, and climbed in behind the wheel. My rhetorical question went unanswered. Required no answer. I had asked it only by way of making conversation anyway.

As I drew up to the post office, Jack stayed me with a hand on my wrist. I glanced at his face and saw not the blank that nowadays was usual but instead an expression of deep concentration.

"Only one," he told me slowly. "'Sovereignty.' You left out the 'i'." I found the error, mid-sentence, page 5, and duly marked in the margin. One misspelled word in 1,200. But he had found it.

29

Although research has come up with better ways to manage and treat the functional ... problems that accompany dementia [Alzheimer's], ... Medicare does not reimburse physicians for the extra time it takes to diagnose and treat Alzheimer's patients.

www.nytimes.com/partners/microsites/
fromcausetocurealzheimers/2.html

Just as some people are born with perfect pitch, others are born with hand and eye coordination that far exceeds ordinary endowment. Jack was one of those. It just came so easily. Hand him a bat, a racquet, or a paddle, and connecting to the ball was second nature.

"You mean like this?" and the ball arcs up and drops cleanly through the basket.

Patiently batting a bucket of tennis balls out to twelve-year-old Mark so he could perfect his fielding technique, one right after another, dead-eye Dick and never missing. He could juggle, too.

Once we were driving in Normandy, calvados country. I was at the wheel and beside me Jack was getting impatient to get wherever it was we were going. He said something that prompted me in a flash of annoyance to gun the car and pass another car just on the brow of a hill. At once, flashing lights behind us. We were pulled over. Papers examined. We were to proceed, staying immediately behind the gendarme's car, to the prefecture where the violation would be more fully explored.

Two Americans, tourists, a rented car, passing on a hill. It made for a nice little drama in the small sleepy room where a handful of gendarmerie lounged, played cards and smoked bales of blue-smoke cigarettes.

I was the culprit. It was foolish, I told the portly magistrate, who frowned and thoughtfully fingered a nicotine-stained mustache. I apologized. I confessed to poor judgment. Ordinarily I was a careful driver. I would not, I assured him, make the same mistake again.

He looked unconvinced. Our two passports were open in front of him. He studied them rather more intently than need required, trying I suppose to figure out what in the world to do with us. Jail overnight? A fine? Suspend my license? Possibly even lock up the passports until some higher authority had been roped into the scene. I watched his face intently to guess his decision. And then, idiotically, a broad smile spread across his plump face. I looked around, bewildered. It was Jack. On the corner of the desk was a blue enamel bowl, filled with small, reddish-green farm apples. Taking three of them, Jack was juggling them in easy, tidy arcs. From the card table in the corner, applause. The magistrate, the better to appreciate the show, removed his glasses and in a moment he too joined in the applause. Smiles all around. I smiled, too. The passports were folded, handed back, and with no further ado beyond a cautionary word to drive please with more care, the door was held open and we were bowed out.

Owen, not quite two, sat on the floor wailing as his mother and father drove away on a short errand. His mouth was a round O of misery. His eyes were dripping bubbles of tears that coursed over fat cheeks and converged in a steady drip at his chin. At once I set to work, more than equal to the task. A shiny spoon and a small kitchen pot to bang on. See!

A blue china rattle that encased a jingle bell. Listen! Peekaboo with a red and white checked napkin. No dice. Inconsolable Owen would sob until his parents returned or until he fell asleep in utter exhaustion. And then Jack stepped in to produce the miracle of three lemons flying toward the ceiling and dropping back safely into his outstretched palm. Again and again. Ah-h-h, the magic of it! Through the tears a four-tooth smile, two up, two down and baby hands delightedly outstretched.

He could juggle us out of a French jail. He could juggle a baby into smiles. He could juggle to make me laugh when I wanted to carp. He could juggle at courtside to pass the time when our game was late in showing up. But now, simple balance was day by day becoming an ever-greater problem.

On a weekend morning Billy showed up, expertly equipped with a level, drill, screwdriver, and a selection of sturdy chrome and white enamel fixtures. With infinite patience he affixed them at crucial spots around the house—at the back steps, near the shower, by the garage door. The work completed, he then, like a good guide, took Jack carefully through the house, placing his hand on each of the new fixtures. "See! Give a tug! It will hold you. So the next time, you come through here, just reach up and grab onto this."

They both were smiling, Jack for the one small extra measure of reassurance, Billy for the pleasure of being able to extend a helpful hand to our beleaguered household. And a helpful hand it was. As Jack would pause, only one small step from his destination, lacking the balance to complete his trip, he would tilt dangerously forward, a trembling hand outstretched. His fingers would curl around that bit of firmly anchored chrome and . . . safety! But short-lived safety.

Early in our second spring. Midday. After lunch Jack lay down to nap and I lay down beside him. I held his hand in mine, staring up at the ceiling in a search of what might await us just around the next bend. I would lay there only briefly, just until he dozed off. I would lay there to rest but not, absolutely not, to sleep.

I struggled back up into wakefulness, sleep-drugged, to hear insistent knocking at the door. Even as I flew to open it I was processing the realization that Jack was no longer in the room.

At the door, a stranger with a kindly face and hesitant manner. Behind him was a car filled with blurry faces. He was just driving down the lane, showing his wife an area where he had once lived. He turned around at the end of our dead-end lane to retrace his route and there, on hands and knees, just by our mailbox, a man, half dressed, who, if he understood correctly, was a resident here? In this house?

No one was hurt. Jack's hands and knees, only minor scrapes. Reassurances came from every quarter. Those things happen, I was told, a generic consolation if ever there was one!

But I was holding onto his hand, I kept repeating to anyone who would listen. I was right there beside him. How could I have been unaware that he was getting up, going outside? I was getting tedious. Besides, it was so obvious—of what use was I if even when I was right there at his side, I was unable to prevent something so potentially dangerous? But of course everyone was too kind to say as much.

*

In the first year of Jack's retirement he was bombarded with what he called "terminal solicitations." They arrived by fax and phone. They filled our roadside mailbox. Did we want a comfortable burial plot? A "family rate" at a crematorium? A bronze urn for the dignified preservation of our cremains? A condo in an assisted living facility with a view of the tenth fairway? A time share in a Florida resort overlooking the shuffleboard court and the heated pool? We also received proposals for every conceivable type of insurance—life, term, dismemberment, accident. Along with all the other gilded offers came multicolored brochures touting the peace of mind that would be ours once we signed up for LTC. Not Loving Tender Care as I presumed, but rather Long-Term Care.

What did we need? What could we afford? What was bogus and what made sense? Finally we gathered them all up, well, not really all, since plenty were sent straight to the trash, and took them to a social services administrator at our local hospital. With the sharp eye of a true pro, she flipped through them, tossing some aside, pausing over others, and coming in short order to rest with a policy that would kick in were we ever in need of at-home nursing care. This, we were told, would, in the long run, be our best bet. Never mind that the premiums struck us as exorbitant. The silky-smooth agent for the policy made short work of such foolish concerns. He pointed out that we would have to be found qualified before we could be swaddled in its benevolence.

Qualified? We thought just being able to write a check that wouldn't bounce would be qualification enough. Not so. Elaborate forms that could only be completed by our family doctor were sent to us. We were quizzed on such matters as our leisure activities, our mental outlook, and our preexisting medical conditions. After several months and considerable correspondence, a letter of congratulations arrived, informing us that we had been accepted for coverage. As Jack so aptly put it, we were now privileged to write out an annual check for a substantial percentage of our income. Good for us!

For several days after Jack was retrieved by the strangers from where he had fallen at the road beside our mailbox, I was paranoid about leaving him unattended, even to go from one room to another. But once again, when confronted with a need to make a major shift in the pattern of our daily lives, the effort seemed just too overwhelming. Maybe with just a bit more vigilance on my part, a repetition could be avoided. To that end I hung a variety of sleigh bells on our doors, not just on the outer doors but on the inner doors as well. Standing in one room and hearing the telltale jingle from another room, I knew at once where Jack was. Like a well-trained sheepdog, I became adept at interpreting every sound, no matter how faint. And for a week or so, I told myself that we were safe. And so we were, provided that I stayed up all night, keeping watch, for Jack was fast becoming a night-walker. Ghostlike, he would wander through the house, restlessly searching, but searching for what? Sometimes I would open my eyes at three or four in the morning to find him quietly getting completely dressed. Gradually it dawned me that another pair of ears, eyes, and hands was what we needed.

And so began a brand new chapter in our lives, a chapter dictated by a succession of exotic names, unfamiliar cooking odors and voices filled with the seductive intonations of the Caribbean, the west coast of Africa, and the rice fields of our own American south. There was Rejoice Amadougou, Elspeth Kimambo, Usayu Soyinka, Meja Mwinge, Praise Bea Anderson—the list went on and on. They arrived at the bus station or the train station, completing a circuitous journey from far-off New York neighborhoods. I would be at curbside to pick them up, fretting at having to leave Jack unattended for the twenty minutes or so that my taxi duties required.

As often as not they came laden with heavy satchels filled with ten-pound bags of rice, with nameless spices folded into small, tidy packets of waxed paper. And almost always they brought a Bible, or paperback edition of the Koran, amply supplemented by leaflets that extolled a Prophet, a Mohammed, the Virgin Mother or a ministry whose appetite for funds was never sated.

Sometimes, though admittedly not often, I wondered what these strangers thought, coming into our quasi-agnostic household, bringing with them all the armaments of faith, a faith that promised glory in an afterlife, respite from care, reward for all their terrestrial toil. It was not a transposition easily accomplished. It was randy old Bobbie Burns who said it best with his famous couplet,

O wad some Pow'r the giftie gie us
To see oursels as others see us!

Once, high in the Indian foothills of the Himalayas, I was the recipient of such a "giftie." I had been given access to the correspondence that passed between a Philadelphian, his Hindu bride, and the family of the bride. The letters were dated 1908 and 1909. Reading one neatly penned letter from the mother of the bride to her daughter, written on the eve of the impending marriage, I came upon a sentence that brought me up short: "It's all but impossible for your Father and me to accept the idea that you plan to bring an eater of flesh into our family."

The phrase struck me as forcefully as a blow. An eater of flesh! Was that how we Westerners were viewed from the other side of the globe? How despised we must be! How scorned by those millions who viewed the morality of their own culture as towering over our own.

Immersed as I was in the complexities of my own life, I was nonetheless struck by the even greater complexities by which the lives of these strangers were bound. In the short ride home I would hear about absentee husbands, abusive or imprisoned boyfriends, drug busts of teenagers, and multiple small children left behind to be cared for by a grandmother, an auntie, a neighbor, and sometimes only by an older child. "How old?" I would ask, and then, when I heard the reply, I'd wish I'd not asked. Eleven or twelve. I would try to imagine leaving my own children at home under comparable circumstance, but I couldn't. It was an exercise in empathy for which I had insufficient strength. Jack was the center, the focus, the nucleus of all my concerns. I had too little left over with which to reassure or comfort this parade of well-intentioned but not-always-helpful strangers. Too little left over to offer children, grandchildren, or friends.

*

The first time it happened, I didn't think of it as a first, to be followed by a second and a third. It was just something that happened, an isolated incident to be dealt with the best way possible. At the time Praise was with us. She had arrived by way of Barbados, Toronto, and Brooklyn. Like the land of her birth, her inner being seemed to bask in permanent sunlight. For every domestic problem she had both a smile and a solution. Or so it seemed. On this particular day she and I together were helping Jack navigate the route from the living room into the bedroom. Praise on one side, I on the other, steering from one safety point to another— the arm of a chair, the back of the sofa, the door frame—careful to keep the in-betweens as short as possible. No more than eight or ten feet lay between where we stood and the bed. Jack stopped, a stricken look on his face. Come on, I urged, just two or three more steps. We're almost there. But we weren't almost there. The two or three more steps could just as well have been twenty or thirty. "I can't, I just can't." And we were nowhere. A chair stood just beyond the reach of my outstretched hand. But at my side, he was sinking—not falling, sinking. We steadied him as gently as we could with all the strength we could muster. Full length he lay on the floor, breathing hard and looking up at us with a half smile, a Don't-worry-I'm-fine expression.

I tucked a pillow under his head, draped a blanket over him, and while he slipped into sleep, Praise and I sat on the bed to consider the next best step. Neither one of us could ever be described as feeble. But our combined strength fell far short of being able to raise a six foot two man from a prone position. With philosophical acceptance Praise advocated "just letting him be." Fine advice for the short term, but not so great for the long term. It was mid-afternoon. Our local emergency squad would not yet be free from their regular work. An ambulance? But ambulances transport people to the hospital and that was one journey we were not about to make. A neighbor? But I couldn't think of any neighbor strong enough to do the job.

So I called Mark.

And calling Mark became the option to which I turned with ever-growing frequency. He lived five miles and four minutes away. He worked his sixty-hour week on the third floor of his house, churning out a nonstop flow of books for junior sports enthusiasts. Our conversations were blessedly simple. "It's your Dad," I'd tell him. "He's down—in the living room, in the bathroom, out on the deck." And always the answer came back, "I'll be right there." There surely were times when my call interrupted a business conversation, dinner with friends, work being rushed through on deadline. But if there were such occasions, they were never mentioned.

With unfailing gentleness, with sure hands and a back of iron, he could lift Jack up and guide him to a safe landing on the bed. But after half a dozen such SOS calls, it was evident that something profound had to change. There were days when Mark had to be away on business. What then? And always I was haunted by the possibility of Jack's not sliding to the floor but crashing. A broken arm, shoulder, hip? If I let my thoughts escape in that direction, the possibilities were truly limitless. Perhaps the time had finally come to check out "an appropriate facility."

30

Medicare doesn't pay for prescription drugs. These drugs are a lifesaver for many Alzheimer's patients because they can keep patients out of hospitals and nursing homes. Many Alzheimer's patients don't get physical, occupational and speech therapy because [of] Medicare regulations.

www.nytimes.com./partners/microsites/
fromcausetocure/alzheimers/2.html

There were two facilities in our immediate community. If Jack couldn't be cared for at home, then surely the next best choice was to have him within easy visiting distance, someplace where family members could stop by on a daily basis.

Mark came with me on that first inspection tour. We pulled up to a large, one-story complex with gleaming glass windows and manicured shrubbery. We were ushered into the director's office, paneled in wood veneer with plenty of artificial ferns to put us at our ease.

The director was so well suited to her role. Middle age and middle management. Everything about her so reassuring—the softly modulated voice, the navy jacket over the pale blue silk blouse with the nicely ruffled jabot. Her head was coiffed in a cap of smartly cut taffy hair with just the slightest hint of gray. Her capable hands were impeccably manicured with a pleasingly pale polish that perfectly matched lips that framed a startling number of white capped teeth. Her smile was broad and on frequent display.

How deftly she dealt with the particulars—name, address, age, physician, date of onset, current capabilities, insurance. What meds are we on now? and I noted with only the mildest interest how that "insider" expression no longer made me wince.

We were complimented on our good judgment in coming over to introduce ourselves. We were told that here our loved one would be assured the very best of care. We were told that once he had "settled in," he would be far less anxious than he was at home. Really?

Such a soothing voice. Listening to its smooth cadences I thought how expertly she would keep us calm when the pilot gave the word to ditch. How, when the earth began to tremble, she would know to stand in a doorway; she would remember that when the car plunged into the canal, you had to wait until the pressure equalized before opening the door. Impossible not to admire the cool competence with which she negotiated the perilous transit along the tightrope stretched taut between professional capability and compassionate concern. No easy feat.

And when I heard myself repeating for the third time that we were only here to "look around," I realized how much better Mrs. Dermonico? Demonica? Mrs. Something, was at handling this whole interview than was I. At least she had a firm grasp on what she was supposed to do. Could I say as much?

The too-sweet smell of air fresheners, the linoleum floors buffed to a gloss, the evident efficiency of the administration offices where state-of-the-art computers blinked tirelessly atop blond oak desks, supervised by a cheery staff in matching pink smocks, the logo, "Caring . . . since 1948" embroidered on the pocket. It all added up to . . . capitulation.

Karen—brisk, reliably cordial, with a cheerleader's build and an engraved lapel pin KAREN, P.N.—was summoned and entrusted with the unenviable task of showing us around. Dutifully we fell into step behind her.

First stop: a "standard room," empty, two beds neatly made up, a wide-armed chair beside a window that overlooked some part of the grounds unseen from the entrance. Peering out I viewed a construction site of some sort where large-wheeled, serious machinery stood idle. The doors of a pair of upright tin lockers were opened for our inspection and we were invited to examine as well the four-drawer dresser: "Two drawers for each of our guests. Of course, we can provide more space if it is requested. But we encourage our guests not to bring more clothing than they will actually need. Our in-house laundry is excellent and we find the provided space is more than adequate."

Any questions? Well, none that I could think of and Mark too came up empty-handed.

So on to The Garden. The upper-case letters were clearly discernible in her buttercup bright voice. We stood, the three of us, in an open doorway, gazing out into an inner courtyard. A bird feeder, a fountain (not turned on), four wooden benches, a criss-cross of cement paths cutting the lifeless grass into quadrants. It was, we were told, "a favorite of our guests." No one was there, but then doubtless this was not the proper hour for visiting The Garden.

Departing the garden we passed a nurse's station where a covey of patients, passive, androgynous, and frail as tissue paper, sat, wheelchair-bound in a semicircle while a nurse presided over a mid-morning repast of fruit juice and crackers. With infinite care she was holding a cup to each one, gently urging small sips, murmuring scraps of encouragement. Several of her charges were secured with obi-like strips of cloth that were firmly tied at the back of the chair. As we passed, one or two briefly glanced our way, expressionless. Not to meet their gaze seemed rude but not as rude as intruding, even with eyes alone, on fellow beings so patently vulnerable. Walking by, I averted my gaze. From some nearby quarter a radio or maybe a CD player was softly playing Judy Garland singing "Somewhere Over the Rainbow." ". . . wa-a-y up high, There's a place that I dream of . . ."

Next came the fitness room. Karen gave a nice little tattoo on the door with her fingernails, flashing us a quick smile. We waited, a trifle too long, and then a robust male "Come in!" We pushed through the door into a modest-sized room where generous windows provided a fine view of the parking lot. A faint and surely forbidden smell of cigarette smoke hung in the air. It smelled good. Never a smoker, I took a good deep breath. It was like breathing in the far-off world beyond these walls.

We were introduced to Michael and Tony, a pair of sturdies and "our resident physical therapists." We all shook hands. We were so pleased to meet each other. We were shown the stationary bike, the treadmill, and a rack of dumbbells, neatly arrayed in order of size. No patients in there either. But then, after all, what did we know about schedules, surely the determinants by which Michael and Tony worked.

So much cordiality. I reminded myself of Marcel Marceau's famous Pip with a smile laminated onto my face—indelible and forever. A slow ache was creeping from my jaws up through my cheeks, locking in around my eyes, and continuing on up into my forehead and my temples.

"Well, great," said Tony when there was nothing much else to say.

"Yes, great!" echoed Michael. Everything was great. It had become our favorite adjective. Tony rubbed two competent hands together in a little display of enthusiasm. "Really looking forward to meeting you folks again," delivered with a smile of undoubted sincerity.

"When did you say Mr. uh . . ."

"Stewart, Mr. Stewart."

"Right! When will he be joining us?"

But learning that nothing was definite in no way dampened their spirits.

"Well, whenever," said Tony.

"You bet," said Michael. And again we all shook hands. Backing out I took one last look, searching for telltale butts. No luck.

As was only proper, the best was saved for last. The dining room. It was a large semicircular room, glass walls, a domed ceiling, and a stage. It was, by any measure, an impressive architectural statement.

"We're very proud of our dining room," Karen told us emphatically and of course we could easily see why. Lunch was evidently being set up. Three or four aides, laughing at some private joke, were laying out silverware at tables for four persons. Our attention was directed to the menu of the day which, we were told, was posted daily. But what was there to say about a fruit cocktail, creamed chicken, rice, and peas, with assorted ice creams for dessert? I would have turned back at that point. But it was evident that Karen wanted to linger a moment or two longer as if to make certain that we absorbed the full impact of the dining room with its lofty dimensions and its stage, so perfectly designed for all manner of entertainment. I knew that simple good manners called for some expression of approval. I searched but came up empty-handed. My entire inventory of compliments had been depleted.

Back to the office for the wrap-up. Any questions? Rising to the challenge, Mark asked if patients could use the fitness room daily, could go out to the garden, weather permitting, daily?

"Certainly! Of course guests who might require assistance are charged what we call an 'excursion fee,' but our whole staff always encourages everyone to use the facilities to the full extent of their capabilities." A few more details—billing, visiting. I only half listened. Despair, bitter-tasting, stubborn, and immune to reason, was building somewhere deep inside me. Like the first intimations of nausea, it blanked out all else. I attempted logic. Why not concede that so much gleaming reassurance, so much undoubted professionalism would, in the long run, best serve Jack's needs? But if that was so incontestable, why was I so resistant? Where was common sense? Certainly nowhere within easy reach.

With a grace for which I was mutely grateful, Mark managed our departure, compensating, or so I hoped, for my own ineptitude.

Much appreciate. Be in touch. Thank you again.

We made it to the door, smiles, handshakes, and yes indeed. "So. Just let us know. We do like twenty-four hours advance notice, whenever possible."

Of course.

The ride home was uneventful. Mark drove. I wept.

31

To be sure, caring for a loved one with Alzheimer's is still a horrific burden for most people—stressful and enormously expensive, with few services covered by insurance.

Claudia Kalb, *Newsweek*, January 31, 2000, p. 52

That inspection trip ushered in a period of ruthless introspection. Friends sought to bolster my outlook with countless anecdotes of beloved relatives who had fared well in the very facility of which I'd taken so dim a view. Nor did I doubt them. Even the harshest critic would concede that well-trained people under the best possible circumstances were doing their utmost to care for people whose conditions demanded superhuman patience and compassion. I saw that. Those artificial ferns, those weights that nobody hefted, those benches on which no one could sit unaided, those smiling, ever-optimistic faces—what after all did I expect? There was no need to remind me that such care was available to only a frighteningly small minority. No need to point out how fortunate we should count ourselves in being able even to consider such care. I knew all that. But still.

Making up my mind not to make up my mind was all I could manage. The idea of handing over Jack's care to an institution, any institution, was a concept I was incapable of accepting. Let's just try to see how we get along. Praise concurred. But neither of us was able to offer a solution to a very basic dilemma, no matter how vigilant we were: Jack's balance was deteriorating at an alarming rate. Every day a crisis or near-crisis. And once Jack was prone, Praise and I together were helpless to lift him up. For that, I had nowhere to turn except to a loving stepson, whose life was being badly disrupted by the ever-present possibility of a phone call, at midday or at midnight, a call to which he never failed to respond with quick reassurance and strength that Praise and I together couldn't begin to match.

For the next several weeks we managed. No more walks to the mailbox. Ever fearful of his falling, I no longer urged excursions in the car. Dinner out at even the nearest waterfront joint, that too was crossed off. With increasing frequency I would put meals on a tray and carry it to the bedside rather than risk escorting Jack from bed to table. With every passing hour I could plainly see how I was inviting the walls to close in on us.

If only, I reasoned, I could find a good strong male version of Praise. Wouldn't that be a solution? I talked it over with the family. Well, maybe, came the response. But how and where was a such a solution to be found? Over a six-month period I had amassed a list of some thirty agencies specializing in providing home care. My search began with the Yellow Pages and branched out from there. I tracked down every referral. No lead, no matter how improbable, was too slim to follow. Meticulously I logged in the date and time of my calls, noting the name of the person with whom I spoke. Noting carefully what I was told. "No one available right now, but if you'll give us a call in a week or so perhaps by then . . ." and in a week to the day, to the hour, I would be back on the phone, tracking down the someone who would enable us to sidestep the decision that loomed so ominously on the horizon.

Finally we came to an impasse. Praise had to depart, summoned back to Barbados by a family crisis that she tried to explain and that I tried to understand. But neither one of us was very successful. Praise said she would return. No, she didn't know when but "as soon as ever I can." Praise had a niece. Would we like to consider having her niece come to help us out?

A niece? How old was the niece?

The niece was nineteen and very strong, very capable. I hesitated. By now Jack was unable to either bathe or dress himself without help, and more help than I, unaided, could provide. Another pair of hands, even untrained hands seemed absolutely essential. How available was the niece?

Praise said she would place a phone call to determine dates and hours. I left the room so she could place the call in privacy. While Jack dozed, exhausted by nothing more strenuous than waking, showering, and having breakfast, I sat beside him, my gaze fixed on the marshland to which life was returning in a burst of springtime exuberance. Green rushes thrusting up through winter-brown bracken, river water on the ebbing tide carrying out shucked off shell and beetle husks—eloquent reminders of nature's irrefutable schedule, predictably unfolding even in the midst of my own irresolution.

I waited for the verdict from Praise. Please, oh please, I intoned, with no idea to whom or to what my entreaty was addressed, let me find a way to keep Jack here in his own house, cared for and cherished in a setting he loved.

Praise returned and with many emphatic nods of her head, with a smile as wide as a sunset, informed me that Evangeline could come. Yes indeed. Would be most pleased to come and would bring Nelson with her.

Nelson?

Yes. Nelson and Evangeline, a two-for-one offer and the expression on Praise's amiable features all but guaranteed the satisfaction of all with any such arrangement.

But Nelson was two and a half months old. He would be no trouble at all, for wasn't he the handsomest child anyone could ever hope to see? A handful of pictures, photographic proof of her assessment, were produced for my benefit, and yes, I had to agree. That infant, fast asleep in the arms of a stout, elderly woman—Grandma? Auntie?—was indeed a splendid specimen of the human race, a roly-poly, freshly minted human being who would require and indeed deserved just as much hands-on care as my beloved, now-enfeebled husband.

For one totally irrational moment I envisioned our household—Jack, Evangeline, Nelson, and me. A quartet of domestic tranquillity. Details to follow. It was a thought that came and went, as evanescent as vapor, leaving in its wake a powerful sense of defeat. Evangeline was not going to wrestle the future into submission.

32

$174,000—The average cost of caring for a person with Alzheimer's throughout the course of the disease.

Newsweek, January 31, 2000, p. 53

Plans proceeded to take Jack for an introductory tour of the facility, which loomed as the next and inevitable step. I suggested the tour to him. He did not acquiesce but nor did he object. It seemed that his illness was consuming an ever-increasing quota of his strength just to exist. It was effort enough with precious little left over for excursions such as I was proposing. In the car he sat with his head tilted back, his eyes closed. From the drawbridge there was a fine view of the ocean, ironed smooth as gray linen with the afternoon sunshine reflecting as from a steel mirror. Deliberately I drove slowly, a senseless effort to forestall completing our mission.

"Do take a look," I urged him. "So calm today, it's a millpond ocean." And he roused himself just enough to turn his head for a long look, a view that when he was well had never failed to delight him, in storm or calm. I slowed almost to a complete stop. He sat motionless, his head turned away from me. I thought perhaps he'd drifted off, but after almost a minute he turned back to me, smiling.

"So beautiful," he told me. When we arrived, several minutes later, I could still detect a glimmer of his smile, a faint trace of lingering pleasure, his memory of the sea not yet eclipsed.

The whole sad business was managed in less than an hour. Introductions, a look at the bedrooms, a smiling, gentle word with the director of nursing, a glimpse of the much-vaunted dining hall, and then, as gracefully as possible, our departure and the drive home.

Finding the right words wasn't easy. Finding any words at all wasn't easy. I listened to myself and heard only irrefutable proof of failure, defeat, and knuckling under, and no argument that really there was no other option in any way convinced me.

"I'm just so afraid of your slipping and falling and maybe cracking a rib or breaking an arm. I think you'll be safer over there. I can come to visit every single day."

I held his hand as tight as I could and as he listened his fingers squeezed mine as if I was the one who needed the reassurance. "It's fine," he said. "It's fine."

Once back at the house he moved as if utterly exhausted. From the car, into the house, and then the long, long journey to his bedside, with each dragging step threatening to be the last step. He fell onto the bed, his eyes closed, and the sleep into which he sank was deep beyond all sight and sound.

That night Billy came, offering more than a strong arm for the ordeal ahead. The actual preparations were simple enough. What does anyone need for a life reduced to bare essentials? I folded and refolded a simple wardrobe. I packed with infinite care the toilet articles that bespoke the entwined intimacies of our married lives. I moved with all the grace of an automaton, laying things with idiotic precision in a duffel bag and then, with the same idiotic precision, removing them all in a mindless search for some small object that had already been accounted for several times over.

Jack was tucked in for the night, or as tucked in as anyone could be who would be up and down a dozen times before morning, when, exhausted and emotionally overwhelmed, I sat down with Billy to a halfhearted dinner. It was late. The leftovers that I shamelessly brought to the table in no way reflected the gratitude I felt for his being with me, compassionate, helpful, and so acutely aware of how I dreaded tomorrow's task. He said all the right things. How would I feel, after all, if in trying to care for Jack at home, he were to fall? His balance was so precarious. An accident could send him back to the hospital and I hadn't forgotten the nightmare of his stay there. If I was relieved of the hour-by-hour caregiving, wasn't it possible that I might even find increased enjoyment out of visiting him? And look how close he'll be, less than six miles away, five point three to be exact.

Billy was so well intentioned. He deserved at the very least some indication that from his words I took some small measure of consolation, of reassurance.

I tried. "You're right, of course," I told him. "Of course, you're right. But still . . ." Not a very convincing performance.

The next morning I took my time fixing breakfast. Like the parent of a birthday child I was at pains to serve Jack's favorites. Grapefruit with just a bit of honey. Oatmeal with brown sugar and milk. A blueberry muffin to go with the coffee. I would have liked the meal to last all the day.

Sitting at the table beside him, I sought to buttress Jack against the enormous change that was about to unfold in his life, and in my own as well.

"You remember where we were the day before yesterday? That place we visited together? After breakfast we're going to move you over there. You'll be so well looked after. I can come every single day. We won't have to worry any more about your taking a header around here, falling down and breaking heaven knows what. It's the best place of its kind and aren't we lucky—it's so nearby!"

No reply.

I tried again. "Mark visited it, too, you know. He agrees that you'll be really better cared for there."

Jack looked up and with an expression of absolute lucidity said, "All this really is is pushing me out of my own house." He said it so calmly, so clearly. So completely without the slightest hint of accusation. It was as if he were simply stating a fact.

At the table Billy, who was standing by to help us with the task of loading up, transporting, unloading, and getting Jack settled, caught his breath. His expression of absolute distress was, I knew, a fair reflection of my own reaction. Was that the truth? Were all these arrangements no more than a pretext to free myself of the hour-to-hour care that Jack required? Maybe I was simply too embroiled in daily minutia to grasp the overall picture. Wasn't Jack's quiet assessment of what we were about to do just one more proof of his God-given ability to cut to the quick of any situation? How many times had I known him to do exactly that, slicing through the chaff of words to find the nugget of truth that others, myself included, overlooked?

I had no proper answer, no rejoinder of reassurance. I cleared away the breakfast debris with arms that felt like lead. To Billy's questions—Shall I carry out these bags? Shall we leave Jeff outside until we get back?—I replied with only a nod, not trusting myself to say a word lest I break down completely, thereby complicating things even further.

We arrived in the late morning. At the door we were welcomed with kindly faces, well-worn phrases of reassurance, promises that all would be well. It just takes a while, we were told. And what could be more reasonable than that?

In the room to which we were shown I busied myself stowing clothes and toilet articles in designated spaces while Jack sat on the edge of his bed, watching me with an abstract expression that gave no hint of his thoughts. Was he fearful at finding himself in these antiseptic, strange surroundings? Did the nonstop procession of unfamiliar faces awaken any anxieties that, were I worth my salt, I should try to allay? My own doubts loomed foremost in my mind. I had so little confidence in what it was we were doing, removing Jack from his much-loved home, bringing him to this place where I'm to believe, must believe, he would be better cared for than he was in his own house with well-intentioned but makeshift assistance.

An electric bell or buzzer sounded. In the corridor a subdued shuffling as those who could walk, started obediently down the hall. Lunch. I was welcome to stay, a small gesture of courtesy for which I expressed only a quick nod though some brief words of thanks were surely called for. At a table for two we sat across from one another, each of us sunk in deep and wholly separate pits of misery. Around us the business of feeding twenty or thirty variously incapacitated men and women—although I noted many more women than men—was unfolding with brisk efficiency. A young man approached, looking official in a white smock and white pants, his face split wide in a grin. Across one arm he held what I mistook for a pile of bath towels. With a quick swooping gesture he plucked what turned out to be an oversized terry cloth bib which he flipped in front of me, deftly knotting the strings behind my neck, managing it all before I could utter a word of protest. He did the same thing to Jack, all the while smiling and crooning an unintelligible litany of nonsense syllables. I looked around and saw the same thing taking place at all the tables. No one objected. We were a roomful of well-behaved children, comfortable in the sure knowledge that we would be properly cared for.

The steamed carrots and broccoli, the slice of meatloaf covered with gravy went largely untouched. Not just my throat but the whole of my gut was knotted tight. The sight of the food and its smell repelled me. A sip or two of water was all I could manage. Across the table Jack's face was pale and drawn with an exquisite fatigue. He stared down at his plate with an utterly blank expression. The clatter of silverware, the sound of plates being shuffled, of trays being set down—the perfectly usual sounds of a dining hall—swam above our heads unheeded. The need to escape it all, to find a refuge, a place of quiet suddenly loomed in the front of my mind with undeniable urgency. I undid the bib and reached for Jack's hand.

"Enough? Shall we go?" And he nodded with unmistakable relief. Together we headed back down the corridor to his room, a journey he was able to manage only by stopping at frequent intervals and resting his shoulder against the wall with closed eyes. An orderly, seeing how depleted he was, passed us, turned back, and laid a steadying arm around Jack's back and guided him to his newly assigned room.

Once in the room, Jack fell onto the bed and was instantly deeply asleep.

"They's most always like that when they first gets here," the man told me. "It's the changeover, doncha know. It takes a while.

But don't you worry, missus. He's gonna do just fine. Just fine." His kindly tone and my own exhaustion came perilously close to dissolving the last of my composure. I laid a grateful hand on his arm, nodded, and made an uncertain way back to the car.

It was as if the very act of consigning Jack into the care of others reinforced my resolve to find a preferable alternative. There had to be a better way. Back at the house I was no sooner in the door than I went at once to check the phone messages, at least a dozen from agencies telling me, No, at the present time we have no male health aides but do keep in touch. And then, a faint ray of hope by way of the final message. It's possible that we might have someone who could be available. Give us a call.

The next three hours passed in a blur of hurried phone calls, I on one line and Marguerite, my blessedly efficient daughter-in-law on another line. First calling the agency and hearing: "We're very sorry, but policy forbids us from giving you the name of the person, but the person will call you."

"But when? How soon?"

"Some time today or tomorrow."

No, no, not today or tomorrow. Right now. As soon as we hang up. Please. Right now!

And then the sitting beside the phone, willing it to ring.

Then, in an incredible reversal of fortune, the phone rang and a hesitant, rather indistinct voice was telling me that, yes, possibly he was available. Exactly when would his service be required? For how long?

I clutched the phone to my ear with the desperation of the condemned one minute before midnight and was this the governor calling?

A muddled exchange of information. His name. Our address. The patient. What was required. When could he come? Could he

33

If current trends continue, Alzheimer's disease will become the epidemic of the 21st century, destroying the lives and savings of 14 million baby boomers and their families. Annual costs are projected to total $3 billion, overwhelming the health care system and bankrupting Medicare and Medicaid.

www.nytimes.com/partners/microsites/fromcausetocure/alzheimers/2.html

The house is still. The late morning sun seeps through the first foliage of spring to etch the lawn with feathery light and ragged shade. Through open windows comes the cold, fresh smell of river water. The air is faintly flavored with onion grass, tangy and knife sharp. Exhausted by the morning's chaos, the hurried, staccato departure from the facility and the triumphant return to home with all its sweet familiarity, Jack is once again in his own bed, sleeping soundly. I pass back and forth through the house, keeping an eye on his unmoving form, relieved beyond all telling to see him there.

Marguerite must leave, tugged back into the complexities of her own life. I fold her briefly into my arms and try to express my gratitude for her presence over the past twenty-four hours.

"Well, we managed, didn't we?" we say to each other, caught up, however briefly, in a sense of euphoria. And oddly enough, neither of us expresses the slightest doubt about Clarence Bell, sitting in there so quietly beside Jack.

She settles in behind the wheel and we exchange one last awkward embrace through the car window.

"My love to the children," I tell her. "And thank Billy for lending you to us."

"Call tonight and tell us how it goes." And I promise.

And one more chapter, hectic, raw-nerved, exhausting, is closing.

Returning indoors I pass the open bedroom door. Purely by chance, the timing is just right: I hover to watch Jack stir, turn, and struggle to a sitting position. Clarence Bell waits, careful not to alarm, and then with infinite dignity, advances, his hand extended.

"My name is Clarence," he says in a voice as soft as woodland moss. "And I'm going to be your friend."

Their hands clasp. Jack nods, his expression totally open, at peace.

"Clarence," he says. "It's a pleasure."

＊

A journey, almost by definition, has a beginning and an end. The beginning is never in doubt. We know the where and when of our starting off. The end we envision, conferring upon it the essentials of time and place. The journey will be short. We prepare accordingly. We carry a minimum of encumbrances. Or the journey will be long and so our preparations must be more elaborate. But rational creatures that we know ourselves to be, we measure, calculate, estimate, and when the moment of departure is at hand, we set off, confident in our preparations.

That spring, the second spring of our new life, I was suffused with the feeling, for reasons impossible to define, that we were poised at a beginning. Life was not to unfold as more of the same. Something behind us had closed. Now the journey will start. But this journey, this final journey, is unlike all the others. The destination is not in question. It is known. It is sure. But the journey from here to there, what of that? Will the way be long? Or brief? I have no way of knowing. I search for signs and find none. What then makes me so certain that this is its beginning? I don't know. But my certainty is huge. Unshakable.

*

Clarence Bell moves into the household as quietly as sunrise and no less welcome. He understands so much without being told. He treats Jack with infinite gentleness but also with amazing strength. From behind the closed door I hear the shower running, the opening and closing of the medicine closet, the off and on splash of the washbasin, the clunk of soap, the click of the Gillette on the basin's rim, and rising and falling, woven in and out of so many homey sounds is Clarence's voice. He croons and chuckles, he sings and speaks, and all of his sounds flow together in a bright rivulet of comfort and caring. Jack's voice, so much deeper, is the punctuation, intermittent but no less essential. It's a duet with each attuned to the other in a kind of wondrous harmony.

Suddenly I am no longer essential to Jack's well-being. Not that I am excluded, shut out. Not at all. I am welcome and welcomed.

"Come here now and sit with Papa Jack," Clarence tells me. "He's been after looking for you ever since he woke." And my reward is the sweetest of smiles from a face too long beset with uncertainty. With a pang I realize what a huge chunk of time has passed since I last saw his features relax into an expression of simple contentment. It's an expression that, for the moment at least, quietly smooths away the heap of niggling concerns that I've taken to hauling around with me, day in, day out.

Who and what was Clarence Bell? The answers came in fragments, sometimes in response to a direct question. Many were offered shyly, even inadvertently, often late at night as we sat together, over a cup of tea, both of us on high alert for any sound from the bedroom where Jack was sleeping.

His story was a facsimile of stories written by tens of thousands of human beings who owe their presence in our midst to our country's longtime, enthusiastic embrace of slavery. How, I wondered, had his forebears come to our shores? He didn't know, though somewhere from out of the mists of childhood recollections he thought there was some familial association with Charleston. Given that city's well-documented affiliation with a slave market that flourished for more than a century, that wisp of childhood memory was doubtless founded on fact.

In stature, tall, slender, light of bone, and dark of skin, he could easily have passed as Senegalese. I had seen what I was certain were his kith and kin, striding the streets of Dakar. Slim and graceful, they wore their long robes with an ineffable dignity, the embroidered caps of Islam on their delicately sculpted heads. The resemblance was too strong to dismiss. But if some antecedent had indeed been captured, shackled, and brought to our shores from west Africa, his name, or maybe hers, had long since vanished. Of his family's history Clarence could go back no further than his grandmother, Ma Goldie Bell of Goldsboro, North Carolina. Of her he recalled only that she chewed tobacco, used snuff, and said she was the mother of his father, James Herbert Bell, who died of drink. Who was her husband? Clarence never knew.

"I'm not sure anyone knew, not even Goldie herself."

Clarence was born in Kinston, North Carolina, the last of twelve children. Ahead of him came Virginia, Willie, Herbert Lee, Helen, Earl, Shirley, Hilda, the twins Donnie and Alina, Regina, and Charles. Somewhere along the way, Willie died.

Of what, I ask.

"Willie just plain died. We never knew why."

Childhood in Kinston meant working the tobacco fields, digging potatoes, weeding and harvesting strawberries, this last a particular favorite because, "sometimes we'd get to keep some."

"What," I asked him late one night, "ever brought you from Kinston to the fringes of New York City?"

"My momma didn't want me doing field work. My sister Virginia, she was the oldest, landed a job up in Elizabeth. She had four children then so my Momma saw it as a good chance for me to get away. So I was sent along with Virginia to take care of her four kids."

The four kids, Janet, Peewee, Piggy, and Joey, were one, two, three, and four years old.

"And how old were you?" I asked him.

"Seven."

When I expressed amazement, not untinged with dismay, that a seven-year-old would be given responsibility for four young children, including a baby not yet old enough even to walk, Clarence only laughed and shrugged it off.

"I didn't mind. Fact of the matter was, I liked being the boss."

Being the boss meant not going to school. He liked that too, at least for a while.

I asked him if he was ever scared, being alone in the house and entrusted with so much responsibility. Remembering how that must have felt, he grinned and told me, "I was little but I pretended I was big. At night, if I was alone with the kids, I'd make them go to sleep, and then when they were asleep, I'd get scared so I'd wake them up again for company."

Clarence made his way through the elementary grades of William Penn School, halfway through Cleveland Junior High and the other half through Lafayette Junior High, and onto Thomas Jefferson High School. Off and on he dropped in and out of various community colleges, working at odd jobs to keep a few dollars in his pocket.

Now he is fully accredited on the bottom rung of our country's health care system. Officially he is a Certified Home Health Aide, a ranking that requires him to attend annual health care refresher courses. He carries an impressive array of credentials that prove he has no criminal record, is free of tuberculosis, has been immunized against rubella and is HIV negative. Today 35,600,000 Americans are 65 or older and by the year 2025 that number will jump to 62,640,000. So we could be forgiven for thinking that Home Health Aides such as Clarence Bell could count on earning not only a living wage but could count as well on certain basics such as health insurance, paid leave, and access to a pension plan. Or so one would think.

But in this, the most powerful nation on earth, health care is totally controlled by the insurance industry. We who were fortunate enough to have secured long-term-care insurance must now proceed exclusively through the channels of that industry if we wish to activate the policy for which we have been paying our annual premiums.

Clarence can work only through state-certified agencies, which places him in households such as ours. Every week his agency bills us. I pay his agency's weekly invoice, a sum in excess of four figures, submitting proof of same to a multibillion dollar insurance company, which, after a wait of eight weeks, reimburses us. Clarence is paid by his agency, which turns over to him less than half of what we were charged. His agency charges time and a half for weekends and double time for major holidays. Yet Clarence is reimbursed at a per diem rate that never reflects either time and a half or double time.

It's a system that is supposed to assure that only crime-free, fully qualified men and women will be hired to care for the sick and ailing. At first glance it might appear cumbersome but reasonably effective. But the second glance reveals a system that shamelessly exploits the Clarence Bells of this world.

Why not hire a Clarence Bell and pay him or her directly? Because our insurance policy dictates that it will reimburse only when services are provided through a state-registered agency. It's a system that is fully entrenched and hugely profitable though precious little of those profits go back to the actual wage earner. Nor are the Clarence Bells of the system provided with health insurance, paid time off, or given access to a retirement plan. Nor will anything change unless and until those same people are organized into a union that can secure for them the pay to which they are entitled, can prevent the agencies through which they obtain employment from siphoning off more than half their wages.

34

Various types of therapy are used to try to stimulate Alzheimer's patients. These include: art therapy, music therapy, playing with toys.

http://news.bbc.co.uk/hienglish/health/medical_notes/a-b/
newsid_439000/439952.stm

That spring and summer I often slipped away, heading just down the road to the beach. In the early morning the eastern sun, pouring in, low and lemony, seemed a reminder, however illusory, of nature's restorative powers. It was my favorite time to swim, before the world really awakened. No sunbathers, no picnickers or beach umbrellas. Just the occasional surf fisherman. From out beyond the breaking line of waves, blinking brine out of my eyes, I would fix my sights on his solitary silhouette. I would watch him wade out to stand knee deep in the surf, so intent, so purposeful. Would watch him arch back and with a flawless, fluid motion, cast his line to Portugal. Treading water, detached and unbound, I sometimes indulged the reawakening of childhood rituals— "Load of hay, Load of hay, Take my wish And roll away"—which was no good unless you then resisted the almighty compulsion to sneak even the briefest glimpse of the passing truck despite tightly squeezed eyelids. "Starlight, star bright, take the wish I wish to-night." My father grew up in the southland and brought to his parental role a thousand superstitions, most of them set in rhyme. Seeing the splash-down of the fisherman's lure meant the wish was granted. Failing to see the splash-down meant wish denied.

But what exactly was the wish?

I never went there. It was too amorphous.

Besides, whenever I lost, I cheated. I'd wait for the next cast. It was two out of three, wasn't it? Or three out of five?

If an early morning swim was out, I'd try to go down at day's end when the foam caught and held the pinks and reds of the setting sun and a wonderful solitude reclaimed the beach. Early morning, early evening, not always, but often enough, I could draw in great draughts of sky and sea and space, all distilled into a wondrous cosmic force that for a moment or two transcended chaos, grief, regret.

The tranquillity that came with swimming, the wonderful freedom of stroking, sliding through translucent green-blue infinity was therapy. But there was therapy, too, in just walking the beach. My ears would fill with the rhythmic suck and surge of the sea. There was odd consolation, reaffirmed with every breath of salty air, in nature's absolute indifference to the human condition. There at the water's edge, Jack's mental deterioration, my own hapless reaction to his decline, was blended into a much broader context that demanded absolute passivity. The arching sky above, the water swirling round my feet, the glare of sun on sand and sea, effectively reduced me to an elemental self. Thought and will suspended. Was that what was meant by an out-of-body experience? Whatever its definition, I welcomed it like a smoker, too long denied, gratefully drawing in the first deep lungful of smoke.

Sometimes friends fell into step beside me, and I swapped solitude for companionship, was nourished by yet another kind of consolation. Always there was something to delight the eye—sand pipers skittering comically ahead of us, gulls diving out beyond the breaking waves, kids sleek as seals racing in and out of the surf. It seemed wholly natural to walk with a friend, sometimes in silence, sometimes not. The kind concern of others did much to offset the tyrannical isolation that Jack's illness had imposed on our lives. How were we managing? Was there anything they could do to ease our situation?

Those walks along the beach, scuffing companionably through ankle deep water, served as an apt reminder that ours was not the only household beset by illness, by disappointment and calamity. In our relatively small community others were randomly struck down, their misfortune sometimes foreseen but usually not. Listening to such distant happenings kindled a sharp desire to be as supportive of family and friends in their particular hour of need as they were in mine. So worthy a sentiment! So seldom realized.

*

Depleted as he was, Jack still clung to shreds of his former self—his love of male companionship and the impersonality that, at least for his generation, was such a trademark of male friendship. The Giants, the Yankees, the latest from the Supreme Court, the success or failure of union-bashing legislation, the follies from the Oval Office—all fair grist for men-only, lunchtime discussion. Safe and sturdy topics and such fine cover for the welcome warmth of comradeship. Now, even though all of that was beyond his grasp, Jack still responded with a kind of mute delight, which was why lunch with Bill was so welcome an event.

The call would come, maybe once a week or every ten days. "How about lunch? Tomorrow? Friday? If Jack feels up to it?" Bill was a much-beloved neighbor and in the days of "before," he and Jack had relished many a meaty discussion on topics of mutual interest. Before his retirement, Bill, a labor lawyer, had been involved in a number of cases that, for one reason or another, had been of concern to Jack. They viewed the world around them with a comfortable commonality. That Bill chose to maintain at least the outward semblance of their friendship was, as I saw it, a gesture of pure compassion. But when I struggled, as I sometimes did, to say as much, to express my gratitude for his generosity of spirit, he would have none of it.

"Not at all," he would say, waving aside my thanks, my appreciation. "I've always loved being with Jack. He's the best of company. We *like* being together. It's my pleasure." As if time and illness counted for nothing.

Bill, driving over to our house to collect Jack for their midday excursion, would be blessedly unaware of the scene that invariably preceded his arrival.

"Bill's coming today. He wants to take you out for lunch. Just the two of you. Maybe at Edie's or that clam hut place you both like so much." It was an announcement I was careful to make not too far in advance lest I plunge us both into a full morning of agitation.

"Who's Bill? I don't know Bill."

For which I was ready with soothing reassurances.

"Sure you do. You and Bill are good friends. Remember last week? He drove you all the way out along the bay? Wasn't that the afternoon of the big thunderstorm? The two of you weathered the downpour and came home to blazing sunshine."

As always I was saying too much, not saying enough, trying with words to blot up, mop up the black vile viscous poison that was seeping through the folds and crevices of his brain. "Bill," I would say ineffectually, a note of far-off desperation drawing stealthily closer. "You'll see, of course you know him, when he gets here you'll see."

"No. No." In a worried tone. "Please. I don't know. Who's Bill?" And the good cheer I was trying so hard to project would only barely keep out ahead of the despair and grief that I could feel, rising behind me in ever-mounting waves.

And sure enough when the moment was at hand, when Bill's hand reached out to take Jack's in his, when he spoke his cheery, "How goes it, my friend?" Jack would smile with a glad warmth of bygone days, would struggle to find the right words, would let himself be helped into the front seat, lifting his hand to me in a jaunty farewell.

It was one of the few rituals left that for Jack acknowledged an existence beyond the parameters of invalidism. Lunch with Bill— always a bright spot in the darkening landscape.

35

Could it really be that patients and doctors alike will come to view Alzheimer's disease in much the same way they now view heart disease— as a serious illness that can be treated and even prevented? That's what Alzheimer's experts are ferverently hoping.

J. Madeleine Nash, *Time Magazine*, July 17, 2000, p. 51

I did all the required reading. I followed the medical bulletins in news magazines, newsletters, and the daily newspapers. I knew by heart all the recommended procedures that every Alzheimer patient should follow: A healthy, nourishing diet. Light on the carbohydrates. Light on fried or fatty foods. No alcohol. Plenty of water. And exercise. Exercise was always emphasized, outdoors when possible, but indoors when the rain poured or the snow blew. We had the one-pound weights. Lift. Extend. Stretch. Lift again even when exhaustion closed down all muscular control. And mental stimulation: Let's not forget mental stimulus. Classical music, books read aloud, word games. The reservoir of helpful suggestions put forth by the experts never ran dry. It all reminded me of a memorable scrap of graffiti, glimpsed long ago on the airline bus running from the Invalides in Paris to Orly Airport. The exuberantly large letters, all uppercase, straggled along the white tile wall of a tunnel. Black paint with only a few drips to suggest that the artist was in a hurry, or maybe only stoned. "TOUT EST PERMIT, RIEN N'EST POSSIBLE." Could anyone have described our situation any better? Je ne pense pas.

In Dr. X's tastefully appointed office we sit alone at a small round table that smells pleasantly of lemon oil. This time we are just two . . . Dr. X and me. My eyes stray to the wall in search of the gray barnyard horse with its laughing rider and its friend, the tagalong dog. But I don't see it. Maybe I'm looking on the wrong wall, even in the wrong room. Maybe I'm mis-remembering. But quickly I rein in *that* line of thought.

This time Jack remains at home. This particular visit has been arranged not at my request but at Dr. X's. It was during a telephone discussion last week that he suggested, not with any urgency but in a pleasant, when-you-have-time manner, that perhaps it would be a good idea for us to set up an appointment in the office " for conferencing," and by now I'm long past letting such semantic absurdities get to me.

Dr. X looks fine. Life in general and evidently this summer in particular are treating him well. As if to emphasize the doctor-to-nonpatient nature of this visit, he has shed his white lab coat and now sits opposite me in a smart tan summer suit. The yellow oxford cloth shirt and dark brown tie with the thin yellow diagonal stripes nicely complete the impression of well being. We begin.

"So how are *you* getting along?" with just the faintest under-
lining of "you." He's letting me know that although Jack is the
patient, I, as the caregiver, must also be considered. It's a relationship that can't be billed and we don't linger there. But isn't
it nice that he detours just enough to let me know he's not unaware that my life may be complicated. Yes, it *is* nice, and I'm not
about to make waves. I tell him, Fine, all things considered, and
he smiles, nods, and now we're both free to get on with matters at
hand.

Placed on the table between us is Jack's folder. Everything is in
there, neatly arranged, chronological order. Page one deals with the
October breakdown that sent Jack to the hospital twenty-two
months ago. Whenever my thoughts stray to those five awful days, I
instinctively recoil, deliberately turning all those recollections aside.
Don't go there. Don't touch. Not yet. And maybe never. Those five
days probably take up half an inch thickness in the file. The next
two inches must include all the pencil-drawn, wobbly clock faces
with the numbers straggling sometimes inside, sometimes outside
the clock's face. Every hesitant repetition or nonrepetition of Tunnel, Apple, Mr. Johnson, and Charity. All of the medications that
have been prescribed, those ongoing, those discontinued, those not
yet tried. Dr. X's general impressions of Jack as to his gait, posture,
reflexes, verbal capabilities, recited into his state-of-the-art office
transmitter and duly transcribed into tidy typewritten reports by the
office staff that sits, sequestered behind plate glass, in full view of
the waiting room—all there in that tidy manila folder.

I wait. Briefly, on my way to this meeting, I indulged myself by
composing my own scenario for what would transpire.

Dr. X would begin, cautious but the barely suppressed excite-
ment seeping into his tone immediately gives him away. "It's still,
you understand, very much in the research phase. Clinical trials

with 1,200 people in Puerto Rico or eighteen people in Milan or 300 in Kyoto, some astonishing results, almost one hundred percent reversals. We're hopeful, even very hopeful. A few side effects, mostly short-term but, and I want to be very open about this, several deaths and as of now no FDA approval. But, given the alternatives, this particular clinical trial—I think you should consider having your husband take part."

Or something like that.

Of course I would say yes. YES. YES!

And not long after, we'd be back in this same office and Dr. X would profess his delight and astonishment. We would never know this was the same man, would we? And Jack would laugh the way he used to laugh. He would stand up straight again, his shuffling gait miraculously replaced by his very own long, quick stride, his firm, sure steps. He'd certainly brush aside Dr. X's cautionary words about "not overdoing it," about getting plenty of rest, exercise, periodic neurological checkups.

Details to come. But the general theme was vivid enough in my head. Only reluctantly did I close it all down.

So how are we getting along? My decision to take Jack home from the facility—any problems there?

He doesn't say, but I sense, or imagine that I sense, a whiff of disapproval. Jack's admittance to the facility was a sad but, let's face it, appropriate, wholly sanctioned way station in the progression of his disease. Taking him out, and so abruptly, and doubtless the details of our hasty, almost furtive departure must all be laid out there in that folder, well, that kind of thing tends to be disruptive. It's not something we see very often. It's not something we'd like to see become. . . . hm-m-m commonplace. The patient's well-being, after all, is our common concern, yours and mine.

But he has no need to lay it all out verbally. I know. He knows. And each of us reads the other's thoughts with ease. We abide by the rules, both of us. He holds his unspoken disapproval delicately balanced against my newly won and very stubborn instincts. We're a good match for one another.

In self-justification I explain Clarence, the level of comfort he's established with Jack, his ability to coax a few extra steps from him each time they walk, arm in arm, on the deck, along the drive. I say I feel that Jack is so much safer with Clarence there, living with us. I say that Jack seems less restless now. More at peace, his agitation somewhat reduced.

Dr. X nods. It's premature, he sees, to disabuse me of this decision to keep Jack at home. He makes a brief note in the chart and then presses on.

Appetite? Sleeplessness? Any increased agitation?

I want to answer in a manner that is both open and helpful. But there is so much about Jack's condition that I'm disinclined to share. So much around which I want to draw a curtain of privacy. All his disabilities. Now just walking from one room to another is a huge task, an impossible task were it not for Clarence. Breakfast. Lunch. Dinner. That trio of once-congenial interludes reduced now to scenes of invalidism as I lift the spoon to his mouth, carefully tipping soup or egg or yogurt between his lips, murmuring inanities that might help keep him awake for just one or two more spoonfuls.

Jack day by day is losing himself in ways I don't divulge. So I don't confide in Dr. X. Instead I recite a litany of tasks accomplished—the weekly trips to the lab for the requisite blood testing. The daily workouts with the one-pound weights. First one arm. Then the other. The summer sun disguising the pallor of his face, my hand on his forearm disguising the ever-growing weakness of sinew and tendon. Yes, we continue the massive daily doses of vitamin E. I've forgotten exactly how vitamin E is supposed to retard the progression of Alzheimer's. It's also possible that in the weeks and months since Dr. X prescribed the 2,000 daily units, vitamin E has been added to the discard pile of tried-but-ineffective medications. Initially promising, ultimately disappointing.

"You asked," Dr. X goes on, "if there was anything new on the horizon." I nod. Yes, I did ask, when he and I were setting up this meeting.

"And is there?" But my very tone gives me away. We both know the answer to that one. Despite my flights of fancy as I drove to his office, I know full well that no miracle awaits. But I'm careful not to suggest by word or gesture that I in any way hold him responsible. Even though I do. Unfair, of course. Unreasonable.

There follows a mini-seminar on what lies just over the horizon for victims of Alzheimer's. Half a dozen pharmaceutical companies are devoting tens of millions to research. Some fascinating genetic work is underway with mice. Support is building slowly, steadily for the beta-amyloid theory, the sticky protein that multiplies incessantly, coating brain cells and rendering them useless. But significant breakthroughs lie just ahead, a very real hope that, maybe even within the next decade, we'll have a handle on Alzheimer's, will be able to control its progress and, in time, even prevent its onset.

Listening, I arrange my face in an attentive expression. I'm reaching for interested, intelligent concern. Like any decent human being I want to convey relief and satisfaction on behalf of future victims, nameless, faceless souls who, thanks to so much pricey work, will, at life's end, not have to shamble off through mental darkness.

I tilt ever so slightly forward to emphasize that he has my full attention. I keep my gaze fixed on Dr. X's not-unpleasing features. In deference to the gravity of our conversation, his brow is indented by a frown, a kindly frown in which I choose to read concern and caring. For an instant I'm distracted by the man's humanity, which so sharply contrasts with my own duplicity. For, in truth, I have not the slightest interest in all those nameless, faceless people who, in some distant future will reap the wondrous benefits of medical research. Since nothing that he's telling me will come to pass in time to help Jack, I am totally uninterested, which only serves to strengthen my determination to look completely absorbed, even nodding slightly at appropriate intervals.

"So now." There's a shift, subtle but definite, from the abstract to the specific, from those hypothetical patients to Jack. "We see a certain course with Alzheimer's, a progression, if you will, that is remarkably similar from case to case."

I nod. The room is air conditioned and until this moment, comfortably so. But suddenly it feels not cool, but cold. The skin along my arms and up my thighs puckers as chills sweep over me. Abruptly I clamp my lips against the urge to let my teeth chatter. I hunch over and wrap my arms around myself to stay warm.

Across from me Dr. X reaches into his jacket pocket and brings forth a mottled green and white marble . . . the big kind . . . the kind we used to call shooters. He places it on the gleaming wood surface between us.

"I often tell my patients that it's not uncommon to see Alzheimer's develop much the way a marble rolls along a smooth surface." He looks up to see if he has my full attention. I meet his gaze, his calm cocoa-colored eyes under pale sun-bleached eyebrows, smooth, flat eyebrows, so different from Jack's dark unkempt eyebrows, as bristly as privet. But I must guard against distraction, so I drop my gaze to the shiny marble poised there between us, a game not quite yet underway. With his forefinger extended, Dr. X holds the marble in place.

"Alzheimer's often goes along like this." With infinite gentleness he sends the marble rolling, slowly toward the table's edge. "And then it drops" and just in time his soap scented hand is there and the marble falls into his open palm.

"Do you see?"

I do.

"The end can come quite abruptly. After months, even years of something close to stabilization."

"And you think Jack's coming . . ." I stumble, searching for the proper words. "You think Jack is, well, close to the edge, is that what you mean?"

"I could be wrong. It's not an exact prognosis. But, the way things are going . . ." His voice trails off and atop Jack's fat folder, his fingers tap gently to some unheard rhythm.

The marble is safely back in his pocket. Briefly I wonder if he always carries it, for demonstrations such as this. Or did he slip it into his pocket just for this, our little meeting here this morning? Are there other uses for that marble? Is it strictly an Alzheimer's marble or is it also useful for schizophrenia, the D.T.'s, for autism, strokes, brain tumors?

I sense that if I'm not careful, matters could easily slide away out of control, so with great deliberation, I push back my chair. I stand up, hand outthrust, and I say all the right things. And Dr. X, in return, says all the right things to me. Shoulder to shoulder we walk to the door. We're two well-behaved, civilized human beings who are doing a fine job of handling a difficult situation with restraint and common sense. I'm proud of both of us. And it occurs to me that Jack, if he knew, if he could know, he also would be pleased. And relieved. He never was one for scenes.

36

By itself, Alzheimer's does not cause death. Most people with Alzheimer's disease die of other conditions such as heart disease or develop pneumonia or other infections.

New York Times Magazine, June 10, 2001, p. 51

In mid-September nature threw a temper tantrum. Hurricane Floyd. Round-the-clock bulletins tracked its trans-Atlantic progress from the Saharan sands to the eastern Caribbean and then north to the Bahamas. Every newscast included details about wind velocity, wave height, and anticipated damage. Weather reduced to . . . or perhaps elevated to . . . entertainment. City dwellers can usually remain aloof to the weather. But situated as we were within easy flooding distance of the river, we maintained an up-close-and-personal relationship with the elements. I suppose because all of his working life had held him city-bound, Jack, upon retirement, had taken outsized delight in the unfolding of the seasons. The departure of the swallows at summer's end, the spring emergence of the snapping turtle from the mud-bottomed pond, the ethereal beauty of the landscape newly draped in snow —he took none of it for granted. Many a house guest had had to endure an animated travelogue by Jack as he spun them around the area, confident that they shared his enthusiasm for an osprey nest, a flotilla of wild swans, or a just-hatched sail-by of baby ducks.

No words of mine could dissuade him. "But maybe they didn't *want* to sit there watching those ducks for twenty minutes. Not everybody is as taken with life in that pond as you are."

"Nonsense! Of course they enjoyed it just as much as I did." And he meant it.

Ordinarily we viewed the arrival of a big storm, be it hurricane or the even more devastating nor'easters, as grand theater. To stand in the dunes watching the fury of a storm-wracked sea carried with it just the tiniest but altogether pleasing frisson of danger. Sure, we were way above the high-water mark. And swaddled as we were in ponchos, scarves, boots, hoods, and sweaters, there was little chance of double pneumonia. It was a kind of elemental pleasure not altogether free of guilt. For here we were, exulting in a spectacle that, either out at sea or along other parts of the coast, would surely reap its quota of human life.

But when Floyd arrived, Jack was well beyond taking any interest. Even on a clear and windless day it was difficult to coax him out of doors. Whether sunshine poured through our windows or whether those same windows were lashed by rain, it mattered to him not at all. Day and night were fusing into a single stretch of faceless time. Waking and sleeping were merging as well. We did our best, Clarence and I, to impose upon him something akin to a normal schedule, though whether it was for his sake or ours was not at all clear.

Floyd was called Category Two. Two among how many? I had no idea.

Our electricity was out, but battery-operated radios reported that north of the Bahamas, waves had crested at fifty feet. As the storm swept toward us up the coast it left in its wake a trail of awesome destruction. In North Carolina the Tar River rose twenty-four feet above flood level, and an official there, with access to the national media, was quoted as saying that nothing since the Civil War had been as destructive to the people of his state. Fourteen inches of rain in twenty-four hours. And Franklin on Virginia's Blackwater River was submerged under twelve feet of water. Twelve feet! Hurricane Floyd, it was safe to say, arrived on our doorstep preceded by first-class publicity.

Ordinarily we would have gone to the beach together, Jack and I. Clearly that was not to be. But something akin to habit still lingered, so late one afternoon, when the storm was at its height, I ventured to the beach for a gull's-eye view.

Head down, hunched against the downpour, I made my way to a high point in the dunes. The thundering of the surf borne on gale-force winds swirled into my head. It seemed almost to swell inside my skull, to pound behind my eyes. The better to breathe, I closed my eyes and took in huge lungfuls of cold and wet and salt. Within moments a frigid damp had sliced through all my layers of waterproof clothes to press against my skin like icy knife blades. My hands, balled tight and thrust deep inside my pockets, felt numb, as useless as stones.

I wanted to walk down across the wind-swirled sand toward the sea but with no hand to hold, no arm to cling to, it was all I could manage just to crouch there, bracing myself into the wind. I didn't tarry.

Carefully, carefully I drove back home, hub-deep along flooded roads. Headlights on, clenching the wheel, I kept on high alert for downed wires and falling limbs. Well before I was safely back in the garage, I came to terms with a simple truth. It was one thing to go storm-watching with Jack. It was quite something else to go solo, on my own. Come the next storm, I told myself, maybe warm and dry at home would not be such a bad idea.

Not too long after the storm, Clarence, Jack, and I made a routine trip, not to the neurologist but to our family doctor. He was someone who, unlike Dr. X, had known Jack "before." That carried a lot of weight with me. He would remember, I was certain, the man that used to be, the tall, strong, energetic person who would turn up for his once-a-year checkup, cheerfully commenting not on his state of health but on the events of the day.

It didn't take long. A bit of poking and prodding, a question here and there, and soon we were seated in the little office being told that all the vital signs were as they should be—blood pressure in the low-normal range, heart was sound, lungs were clear—and he was pronounced infection-free. Why then had he lost more than twenty pounds since our last visit just a couple of months before? Why was he so obviously sliding down some steep incline toward incoherence, immobility, and unawareness?

"Keep in touch," I was told as we departed. "If you need me, I'm here." Words that offered no holding back of what lay ahead, but words that nonetheless, if even for the instant, were hugely comforting.

Not long afterward, from a kind friend I secured a wheelchair. The first few days it was only an accessory, a gadget reserved for major excursions in the driveway. Before the week was out it had slid into daily use. Life was becomingly frighteningly simple. Even meals that had provided small, not unpleasant breaks in a featureless day, were gradually reduced. Favorite dishes were sampled, then set aside. The autumn was unseasonably warm, but Jack was never warm enough.

The past year had sharpened my skills in providing Jack with whatever phrase or word that eluded him. "I need . . . I need . . ." and when I could say "Your cap? The mail? Your glasses?" my reward, so gratifying, though bestowed for but an instant, was his expression of huge relief. But day by day my word-producing talents were of less and less use. The angst that seized him when a phrase, a name, an object hovered just beyond his verbal grasp eased away. Some time when I wasn't noticing, he ceased to grope for the elusive. Speech dwindled into inchoate sounds and his needs, whatever they were, were left to Clarence and me to anticipate and provide.

Alzheimer's is known, even among the medically illiterate, as the "forgetting disease." The victim's past drifts away. Names, faces, events blur and slowly, or maybe not so slowly, vanish. It's a phenomenon that's endlessly described at every level of accessibility from supermarket tabloids to medical newsletters. But no mention is made of the fact that not just the past but also the future vanishes as well. For Jack, tomorrow disappeared as irrevocably as yesterday. I tried, without success, to imagine life in which both past and future were nonexistent. To imagine one's self locked solely into the Now, nothing in front, nothing behind. It was an exercise that generated such an overpowering sense of suffocation as could only be dissipated by some immediate physical activity—a frenetic burst of weed-pulling, leaf-raking, or floor scrubbing.

By early November I was sharing the Now with Jack by sitting with him, my hand in his, reading aloud whatever book I happened to have at the moment. No matter the subject. He listened or didn't listen, his eyes open but more often closed. But if I stopped, his expression would change. He'd look at me, something akin to a question in his eyes, and only when I resumed reading would he relax again.

Throughout his illness we had maintained the trappings of normalcy—rising at a respectable morning hour, bathing, dressing, meals at reasonable intervals, exercise and rest punctuating the hours until evening brought release and his exhausted return to bed, that blessed bed. As tempting the prospect of remaining all day in bed, it was a prospect sternly resisted. No day passed in pajamas or dressing gown. No meals were brought to the bedside. It was as if by a routine of determined normalcy, the progressive nature of the illness could be held at bay. But as the days shortened and the nights lengthened, that well-grooved routine began to fray. Even Clarence's most compelling persuasion was insufficient to move Jack into the wheelchair for the briefest of excursions.

Wheeled to the table, he had neither interest nor appetite. I would sit beside him, intent on getting a few spoonfuls of nourishment past his lips. With a gesture of infinite patience, Jack would lift his hand to gently deflect the spoon. A sip of water or milk but not much more was all that could be managed.

On the third or fourth such evening I appealed to Clarence. "Not even water," I said, "or milk or soup. If he doesn't eat . . ."

"But don't you see," Clarence told me, "he don't need it no more. He's doing what he has to do."

The marble had reached the table's edge.

The end when it came was so gradual that life would have slipped unremarked into death had we not been keeping vigil. It was his second full day of staying abed, sometimes awake but more often asleep. Mark stopped by not once but twice. When Jack made no gesture to acknowledge his presence I said, and I think I really believed it, "Tomorrow. He's just been very tired today."

That morning Cathy telephoned for an update. I told her almost the same thing. "No, don't come today. He seems so worn out. But if you come tomorrow he'll surely be more alert."

We held a long moment of silence between us and then she said, "I'm coming today," my protests all unheeded.

That night the moon was full. It rose red-gold from the eastern horizon, improbably huge, paling as it made its slow ascent. From a cloudless sky it poured down, bleaching to a milky white the marsh and river beyond. From a chair beside Jack's bed I gazed out across a wondrously luminous landscape.

I both knew and didn't know, accepted and denied. How often in the recent few weeks had I asked myself, would I really want him to stay? Would I really want to hold him in this state of nonbeing, he who had been so vibrant in the fullness of his life? But each time I asked the question, it's not without shame that I say my answer was never a straightforward No. Did I really think that life with only the shadow of the man I loved was preferable to life without that shadow? Even today, I'm not really sure.

It was Clarence who knew when Jack's heart took its final thump. "Just give us a few minutes," he told me, "and then we'll be ready."

So we waited, Cathy and I, standing outside the bedroom, our arms wrapped tightly around each other, providing the few moments of privacy that Clarence requested. Then summoned, we returned to the bedside where all was in order, Jack's long, once-powerful body making too insignificant a heap beneath the blankets.

I turned the bedside light off and let my eyes adjust. The first and sudden darkness melted away. Through the windows moonlight flooded the bed, its pillows, and Jack's face. By its ethereal light his features in death looked more familiar than they had for many weeks gone by.

There were things to do, calls to make, details that must be dealt with. But above all else I wanted only to stand there in the moonlight, not speaking, not moving. I had the odd conviction that if I could keep myself centered in the moment, I could hold time at bay. Up ahead lay all the grieving, waiting to receive me. But please, not quite yet.

I drew the covers up over Jack's hands. They still felt warm, warmer than my own. This was the moment I had so often visited in my imagination. Now those imagined moments seemed infinitely more accessible than the moment at hand. I wanted to embrace regret, relief, and a longing for what would never be again. I wanted to be as one with the essence of who Jack was. But instead I was aware only of a great diminishing. He was gone. And so, I felt, was I.

EPILOGUE

His had been a journey across dark, uncharted seas. Once underway there was no safe harbor, no returning to home port. There was no hope of rescue. Alzheimer's is a one-way voyage to be navigated without benefit of map or compass. For some the journey is cruelly long. For the fortunate it is blessedly brief. Jack was one of the fortunate.

*

It was early, early on a truly perfect summer morning. Mark, Jenny, and I went down to the ocean's edge before the world was astir. Not a soul in sight. The sun, freshly rinsed by the sea, laid golden light across the water. It turned the foam to iridescent crescents, carried toward us by glassy waves. The August air was warm, not yet hot, and a light breeze stirred at our backs. We shucked off our shoes and waded out and then each of us took turns scattering the fine granules that were Jack's ashes into the aqueous light. It was just as it should have been, just the three of us, the three who loved him best. No minister, no prayers, no hymns, no weeping. Just the perfect summer morning, the sea, the light, and the dust rising and drifting out over the water. It felt so exactly right. It took but a handful of minutes. And then we embraced.